That Skinny Girl Life

A life that many women literally want to live

By Alison Jake

Published by: Exhilarate Publishing in USA

Cover Design by Riyana Shami

First page of chapter drawings creator: Shalini Saha

ISBN-13: 978-0692503041 (Custom Universal)

ISBN-10: 0692503048

TABLE OF CONTENTS

Acknowledgements

Before writing this book, I was nervous about sharing my story. I was encouraged to write this book by those who came to me with compliments and questions. My aim was to obtain all the information I need to be able to assist others. With all the diet-books and quick weight-loss regimens in the market, I asked myself how my book would stand out from the rest. I learned that people are desperately searching for hope and are hungry for success stories. I'm a firm believer in proper planning, conscientious eating, exercise and discipline. Everything I have achieved in life is due to hard work and perseverance. There are no shortcuts and nothing is wasted.

I am extremely grateful to the group of people who have continuously asked me to share how I maintained a skinny body and healthy lifestyle. I also want to thank the doctors and nurses who have assisted me by answering my questions while writing this book. I wish to send my good thoughts and appreciation to the people who have trusted me with my advice and support. I have come a long way with all the knowledge, I've acquired, but this book wouldn't exist without all your support, so I thank you all for that.

Writing this book proved to be one of the best investments of my time and mission. Building relationships with others and being able to give my perspective has assisted me in writing That Skinny Girl Life. Writing this book has inspired me to share my Story with my readers.

My goal is to provide hope to each one of you. Please join me in reaching as many readers as possible. Thank you for all your time and support.

Who I Am

Over my lifetime, I have been plagued with questions about how I stay so thin. No matter where I go, whether it's a clothing store, grocery store, or anywhere out in public, people often ask me how I stay so thin. Answering these questions over and over is one of the reasons I chose to write this book.

But before diving into my theories, advice and opinions on how to lose weight, I would first like to tell you a little bit about me.

First and foremost, I am not a dietician, doctor or a fitness trainer. I am simply someone who wants to impart my knowledge of how I manage to stay thin.

After the questions came repeatedly, I began to wonder why people would ask. Were they merely giving a compliment in the form of a question, or could it be that they really wanted to know? Did they really want advice on how to become and stay thin?

If I wanted to know how to do something, I think it is sensible to ask and take advice from someone who has done it. So perhaps these people just wanted to ask how to be thin from someone who has been naturally thin and relatively healthy her whole life. Wouldn't you want to know this valuable information too? Yes? If this is the case, what better person could you ask, other than the healthy, skinny girl herself? Sounds reasonable, right?

After thinking about all of this: the questions about being thin, considering why people would ask, and determining my own opinions, I decided to write this book. I have heard of or met, countless overweight women who are on a diet right now, trying to lose weight and struggling to become skinnier. There is nothing shameful about that. They've tried numerous diets and ideas on how to lose weight, but have failed. In my opinion, if you want to become a skinny girl, you first have to learn what it takes to be one. I decided I wanted to answer these questions on a larger scale by writing this book and sharing it with woman everywhere.

INTRODUCTION

It seems each year we hear about more Americans becoming overweight or obese. It also seems as a nation, we are beginning to view being overweight as the new norm. After all, everyone around us is the same overweight person—so it must be okay—right?

If being overweight starts to become the norm in America, and people do not care about the fact that it is unhealthy, then this view can and will damage the American society as a whole. We will continue to eat in excess and our health will decline, making healthcare costs skyrocket.

The government and various organizations are trying to decrease obesity rates in America, but it does not seem to be working. Why? Are people simply not listening or is the information not being provided in a way that is easy to understand?

In America, we are the land of excess. We want more for our buck and having more of everything is a good thing, but can it be too much? Although we love to live in excess, Americans also spend more money annually on diets and health-food products than in many other countries. It seems to be an odd dichotomy. We want to have our cake and eat it too. However, diets are typically just quick fixes—not long-term solutions.

What is the solution? How do we determine what a healthy weight is, what foods are truly right for us, and how we can best make our own decisions?

As a skinny girl my entire life, I've learned the pros and cons to leading an excess life. I've learned what works best for me and how to determine my healthiest weight. It's a simple solution of thinking your way thin in order to change your lifestyle and obtain your skinny girl self.

That Skinny Girl Life contains research, advice and my opinions about what factors have contributed to this new "norm," why Americans have trouble losing weight (and how major

Corporations contribute to that obesity), and what we can do to reverse these trends. It all starts with what we eat and how we eat too much. Let's get started.

CHAPTER ONE: What It Takes To Be A Skinny Girl

From one woman to another, there are a lot of misconceptions about what a skinny woman does to remain skinny. In this chapter we'll talk about the myths of eating healthy and how to balance the how with the what. We'll discuss the issues of calories, quality versus quantity, and living a torture free life.

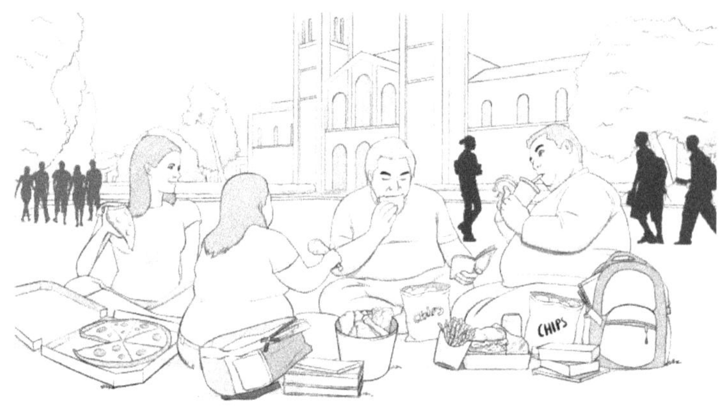

Avoiding the Freshman 15 and still be "unhealthy"

Occasionally, throughout my childhood, I was told by doctors that I had low iron in my blood, which was mainly caused by my diet. This meant nothing to me as a child except that my diet was supplemented by iron pills to help my body with this necessary nutrient. Although I was eating well at home, I wasn't eating enough iron rich foods like green leafy vegetables. Let's be honest… there were green leafy vegetables present at every meal, but what child eats leafy green veggies?

When I entered college, I started living on junk food like beefy, cheesy nachos; saucy, spicy wings; salty potato chips dunked in all sorts of creamy dips; and a variety of the local fast food fare. It was convenient, I had no one to make me home-cooked (or healthy) meals, and of course, it was tasty. Who doesn't love a salty, greasy plate of nachos on a Friday night after a particularly hard week of classes and exams? Like my childhood leading up to this point, I ate what a normal kid would eat—despite it not being the healthiest option.

Despite eating all this unhealthy (and yet tasty) food, I still didn't gain the legendary "freshmen fifteen," nor did I become overweight. How was that possible? One answer is that while I ate all this unhealthy junk food, I only ate it in small portions. Instead of only filling up on these greasy, nasty foods, I utilized vitamin supplements and nutritious drinks to complete my diet. I witnessed a variety of students around me eating the same things I was (minus the vitamins and drinks), but in much larger quantities. Every time I went out with friends they would ingest super-size-type value meals while I would only get the single burger. Or they would get a whole plate of those delicious nachos for themselves, while I chose to split mine with a friend.

They all gained significant weight, while I did not. It was not difficult to make the connection in the differences. Soon my theory developed: “It’s not about *what* you eat, but about *how* much of it you eat.”

Despite not gaining weight, I knew the foods I was eating would eventually damage my health in the long-term. That’s why I started taking vitamin supplements and drinking healthy drinks to gain the nutrients that the oh-so-tasty (but oh-so-not-nutritious) fast food and junk food lacked. I truly thought I had it all figured out! I could eat my cheesy nachos and have my health too!

One day, I made a doctor’s appointment to have a regular checkup, and they tested my iron levels (just to prove to myself that I was making smart choices). Up until this point in my life, I assumed that just having good iron levels would make me a healthy individual. Iron, a mineral found in our blood, acts like a little train for our oxygen—helping it to get from one place to another in our bodies. Without enough oxygen, our bodies can become fatigued quickly and can impair our ability to do work. This certainly wasn't something I wanted to happen during my college years—I needed all the energy I could get!

When I sat down to talk to the doctor, I expected to hear the news that my iron was low due to my "poor" diet and that I would need to take iron pills again. To my surprise, the answer was not the one I'd expected. The doctor said that my iron level was good.

How had my iron level become good suddenly? And was this the reason that I wasn't gaining the weight of my friends? Then I realized my iron levels may have been the result of the vitamin supplements and nutritious drinks I'd been consuming. Even though my iron level was where it needed to be and I wasn't considered unhealthy yet, I still knew that my unhealthy eating habits would eventually catch up to me if I didn't stop them now. Although the drinks and vitamins helped me out for the short-term; they put me somewhere between "healthy" skinny and "unhealthy" skinny.

"Healthy" skinny involves eating nutritious foods (not just supplements) and providing your body with a balanced diet, which even includes healthy fats and carbohydrates. "Unhealthy" skinny can be achieved by simply robbing your body of the proper food and nutrients it needs, or by eating very tiny portions and supplementing with vitamins.

I was somewhere in-between, because I was providing my body with fats and carbs (just not really the good kinds) as well as supporting it with nutrients (compliments of my vitamins and health drinks.) But vitamins and health-food drinks could not sustain me forever (contradictory to what many "health-food" companies will tell you) so I decided to start eating healthier (via good grains and vegetables), cutting out the fast foods and junk, and made the transition to foods that would sustain me and my health for my future.

I also started thinking about what would increase my overall health and what it meant to maintain it.

The BMI and other healthy qualifiers

Ever heard of the BMI? It's your body mass index and is frequently used to determine how healthy you are based on your mass and height. While this is a good indicator of your health and weight, there are regularly cases when the BMI does not apply. Many critics claim that the BMI does not accurately factor in how "healthy" a person may be. For instance, muscular people often weigh more than the BMI suggests. This is because muscle mass adds weight to their frame, but this obviously doesn't mean they are unhealthy. Different countries also have different variations of the BMI scale. Japan does not have an "overweight" classification like the US—only "Low," "Normal," and "Obese." So while you may be considered "Normal" with a BMI of 25 in the US—you would be considered "Obese" in Japan!

The World Health Organization considers a BMI of less than 18.5 to be severely underweight and may even indicate an eating disorder. Different countries have different attitudes, however, about what is considered "skinny." Someone from an another country may seem severely thin with the personal attitudes of the American public, while someone from another country may feel that most of Americans seem quite overweight—even obese.

Although the BMI is used by governments and medical facilities in quantifying your overall "health," what you eat is probably the best way of charting your own course with your diet. Determining what can be called "healthy" foods is often a guessing game for most people (much like trying to figure out the BMI scale!), but sticking with natural fruits, vegetables (especially the green leafy kinds like kale), and whole grain products are a good start. Adding in grass-fed poultry and fish augments the health benefits. Dairy can also be a good source of dietary intake, but be careful of the fat. Whole milks and cheeses can contain more fat than is healthy for a normal sedentary person, so be sure to opt for alternative forms like soy or skim. There are a ton of alternatives on the market now for dairy products—pick something that you like, but do your research on its actual health benefits.

Candy, doughnuts, pies, cakes, sugary sodas, fried foods, some types of "fruit" juices, snacks and that super-sized value meal at your favorite fast-food place frequently creep into our everyday nutrition when our time is short and our energy is low. I almost fell into this exact pattern during my college years. These quick "pick-me-ups" are really just a recipe for disaster, as many of my friends found after they gained so much weight. These foods give you that quick sugar high—which seems like energy—but in the end, you crash and just need more of these "quick fix" foods to keep going.

Even though most of us crave these types of sugary goodies and fast-food indulgences, they have little to no nutritional value and are actually just empty calorie foods. This is why I initially began supplementing with the vitamins and health food drinks (thinking I was being smarter than my fellow college students!) Even though we're adding calories—and it feels like we are full and have energy—we aren't adding substance. My vitamins and nutritional drinks gave me a dose of the nutrients I needed, but I was still verging on "unhealthy" skinny because I wasn't getting those nutrients from the right sources.

I'm not saying what you eat doesn't make you overweight. Obviously eating candy, donuts and fast food ONLY will make you an overweight and unhealthy person. (Again, this is why I was so close to the edge of what was considered "unhealthy" and why my friends gained weight.) But that it is not the case ALL of the time. It's more about how much food, the amount you consume, and how many calories you take in, that makes you overweight. There needs to be a healthy balance to every aspect of your eating habits.

Quality versus Quantity

So let's get back to my theory: *what* you eat versus *how* much you eat. It really comes down to *Quality* versus *Quantity*. Eating a large quantity of food, no matter what the quality, will definitely lead to being overweight because, healthy food or not, a person has to consume more calories than the body uses up in a day. So eating a large quantity of healthy foods, but having a sedate lifestyle, can also have this affect.

Eating mostly unhealthy, empty calorie foods will eventually make you unhealthy, even if the consumption is in small quantities. There needs to be an overall balance to what and how much you eat. Your diet should mainly consist of healthy food with snacks and sweets on the side as treats and rewards and stay within the normal caloric range for your body per day. So what's a "normal" calorie range, you say? Let's have a look.

Calories Do Count.

Have you ever watched a TV program that showed someone who was morbidly obese? A morbidly obese person is someone who is drastically over their recommended weight limit and generally has trouble moving because of their bulk.

Let's look at an example. A twenty-five year old woman of average height and weight needs roughly 1500-2000 calories a day to maintain her weight. The morbidly obese woman would need around 3000 to maintain. But many of these obese people had been consuming up to 5,000 calories *a meal*! I can recall one woman stating that for her breakfast she ate what an average person would eat in two days. Can you imagine eating almost one week's worth of food in *one day*? For every 3500 calories a person consumes above what your body needs, they will gain a pound. You do the math.

One woman stated that she consumed around 34,000 calories a day. That is enough calories to feed seventeen adults in one day. Other people mentioned that they would eat a whole carton of eggs, with other foods, just for breakfast. In addition to the massive caloric intake, these individuals spend at least $200 to $500 a day on food. This becomes not only a detriment to their health, but also to their wallets! These people are literally eating themselves to death.

One thing to keep in mind is that morbidly obese people also add many healthy foods to their diets. However, they eat such a large amount of food in general that it still becomes unhealthy. This takes me back to my theory: "It's not about *what* you eat, but *how* much of it you eat." Once the morbidly obese individual gets to the point that they want to start eating healthier to lose weight, they need to work with doctors and nutritionists to start down the healthy road. Simply cutting massive amounts of calories could also be detrimental to their health. This is why it's important to make changes before it gets to this point.

Some people believe that if you eat a lot of healthy foods, or just strictly healthy foods, then you will lose weight. Such individuals will eat 2,000 calories of healthy foods a day, expecting to drop those extra pounds. After all—it's healthy so therefore, I'll be healthy. But I believe a person can become overweight just by eating healthy foods, if they consume more than they burn off during a day. For example, if a woman eats more than 2,000 calories worth of fruits, vegetables and other healthy foods during the day and is not burning off the excess calories, then she can gain weight from those extra calories—no matter what kind of food makes up this caloric intake. So it wouldn't matter if I just ate the same calories in healthy foods as

I did on all those unhealthy foods—I'd still probably gain weight.

Time for an example: A woman, who is considered "skinny" according to the BMI scale, eats only apples, whole grains and vegetables every day. She'll maintain her healthy weight then, right? Not necessarily. What if she eats 100 apples a day and five loaves of whole grain bread? Seems a bit excessive wouldn't you agree? But it's all healthy foods—just too much of it. She won't be able to sustain this caloric intake for long before adding weight to her frame.

Exercise is obviously an important key too—one we'll discuss in subsequent chapters—but in summary just remember: to become a healthy skinny person, you have to eat like one. Which includes making every calorie count.

Skinny Girl Meal Patterns

For women, how they eat is just as important as what they eat, but there is no ONE pattern for eating a skinny girl way.

First, in our fast –paced worlds, many people skip meals during the day. I was certainly doing this in college as I was trying to keep up with my demanding schedule. Long gone are the days of three balanced meals a day around the family table. People simply don't have the time to sit down and enjoy those three meals. So they may skip breakfast, lunch or dinner. So one type of skinny girl may be on the go until they have time for the next "balanced" meal, and they supplement with protein bars, on-the-go snacks and, sometimes, not-so-healthy sugary drinks.

Here's an example: Perhaps Ms. Skinny Girl Professional needs a little something to eat before heading into that big meeting with the boss and she has only ten minutes. She might pick up an apple and a piece of low fat cheese to get her by.

Maybe she was too busy getting the kids out the door this morning so she had to sacrifice her own breakfast in the process, snacking on a whole grain bagel while in the car instead.

The meal people skip the most is breakfast. One of the most common excuses is that they didn't have enough time. Others claim that they did not wake up early enough, or they were simply not hungry. But this may just be the way they choose to eat. This is their meal plan.

Secondly, some skinny girls may eat three meals a day, but they are smaller and lighter than a regular meal. For example, our professional woman may eat one fried egg, two strips of bacon and a glass of orange juice for breakfast. She may eat a sandwich, a handful of chips, and maybe a soda for lunch. Finally, she may eat a piece of chicken along with mashed potatoes and steamed vegetables for dinner. This may work for some people and can lead to healthier eating habits and lifestyle. But someone who eats all three meals a day could also have the tendency to overeat as well—causing weight gain. It's all a personal choice – you must choose what works best for you.

The third way that a skinny girl may eat is to eat three full meals a day, and also move around a lot, or exercise a lot, so weight gain is avoided. When I mention that skinny people may move around a lot, I don't mean your typical gym workout routine. There are other ways people exercise other than the traditional ways. Perhaps their jobs require a lot of walking or even running errands. College students know this lifestyle—running off to classes constantly. The more a body is on the move—the more calories they are burning throughout the day. Some stay-at-home women especially keep themselves busy with household chores like cooking and cleaning. Moms also tend to be more on the go with children they need to keep up with.

The fourth way a skinny girl may eat is by using a combination of the three ways mentioned above. They may eat three light meals one day and then the next day they might eat only one or two meals, sometimes with snacks between. Some may even utilize a cheat day. This is something some skinny people may utilize on a weekend after a week of very healthy eating. Perhaps they skipped a few meals even to make up for the extra caloric intake of the cheat meal—trying to keep their overall calorie intake for the week to a certain level.

Additional Points to Ponder

One of the main reasons some skinny women eat a small amount of food is that their stomachs can only hold so much. This may lead to the question of how skinny women become overweight, since their stomachs will only handle so much. The answer to that is that they will start to overeat for various reasons--social eating is one, to finish off a plate or not to waste food is another. The more you eat the more your stomach grows to house the extra food thus enabling the once skinny women to now become overweight. Such women will force themselves to eat more than their stomachs can handle. Over time, the extra food causes the stomach to grow to accommodate more food. The more you eat, the higher are your chances of gaining weight.

Despite the different ways skinny women eat, there are still some who claim they eat a lot of food but don't gain weight because of their metabolism. While I do agree that metabolism may play a role in losing or maintaining weight, metabolism is shown to slow down as we age so they won't be able to rely on this forever.

Starting off with a balanced, healthy plan for eating and exercise is truly the only way to maintain a healthy lifestyle over the course of your whole life.

Don’t torture yourself.

The number one mistake people make in their diets is torture themselves. People will eliminate the foods they like from their diets and try to force themselves into eating only foods that they wouldn’t normally consume. For instance, a woman may truly love and enjoy eating spaghetti, but has been led to assume that those heavy carbs are making her fat. So she cuts out the meal altogether and robs herself of that joy. A better solution would be to substitute whole wheat spaghetti for the regular noodles or simply cut back on her portion size. A woman may get rid of all the sweets in her diet and try to only eat healthy foods. Now instead of snacking on the sugary goodness of a cream-filled donut she’s eating an apple instead. It just isn’t the same no matter how you slice it. While it is good to eat healthy food, even if you don’t like it, the most important thing is to not make it the main part of your diet. Choose foods that you like and are healthy. In this instance, maybe a cup of pudding would satisfy her craving for the creamy filling.

I like a lot of healthy foods, but not too many green vegetables so I tend to avoid those because, to me, it feels like torture. I often choose the greasy, fried and sometimes sugar-loaded unhealthy foods over the healthier alternatives. I think they taste better, and it doesn't help that they are also more addictive. One thing I've tried with these greasy, fried foods is to try them baked. You'd be surprised how similar they are and the calories are cut significantly.

In addition, you never want to get rid of sweets completely, unless you know you can handle it. It is okay to eat sweets now and then to reward yourself. This can also encourage and motivate you to continue your diet. Just reduce the amount you're eating. Skinny girls eat sweets, too, and it doesn't affect their weight much. If you get rid of all the foods that you enjoy, it may cause you to go off your diet. Eventually, your diet will fail, because most people are not going to continue doing something they don't like. Eating should not be tortuous—find ways to eat what you love in a more healthy way.

CHAPTER TWO: EXERCISING FROM A SKINNY GIRL'S PERSPECTIVE

Exercise doesn't have to be boring, but it does have to happen. Many skinny girls know this and have many tips and tricks that help to keep them on track and keep fighting fat. In this chapter, we'll find your exercising style, give motivational tips, and provide information on why fat slows you down.

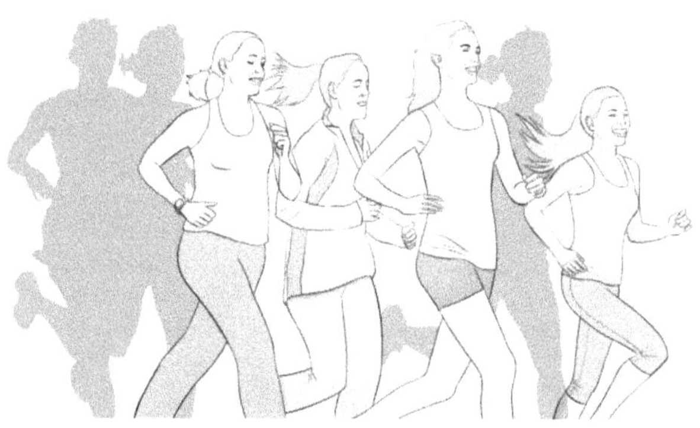

Get out of that stinking gym

I mentioned exercise earlier as an asset to losing weight more efficiently. The definition of exercise, according to TheFreeDictionary.com, is "*an activity that requires physical or mental exertion, especially when performed to develop or maintain fitness"* and is *"physical exertion, especially for the purpose of development, training, or keeping fit."* Another way to define exercise is to think of it as anything actively physical that gets your heart pounding and blood pumping. For some, this could mean a simple, fast walk and for others it could be the popular Zumba (which we'll discuss later in this chapter) or even a dance class.

To many people, exercise is moving your body in a way that benefits you, such as helping you to build muscle mass, lose weight, or tone up, but for many, the word "exercise" is a nasty word. It brings up images of excessive sweating, sore muscles and endless hours at a smelly gym.

Skinny girls don't always go to the gym and exercise. I've known a few skinny girls who do a lot of couch sitting as their "exercise!" The skinny couch potatoes are most likely not eating that much food to gain weight, and that's why they're still skinny. Maybe they have a great natural metabolism or maybe they eat just enough to maintain the weight they have. You see, even if you're not moving a lot during the day, your body still expends energy from the simple things like getting out of bed, taking a shower and even eating. Your body knows the exact amount of calories needed to maintain your weight doing only those activities. If you just eat that many calories, you will neither lose nor gain any weight. This is often how a skinny girl can do no exercise and still maintain her skinny status.

On the other hand, some skinny girls just love to work out and be active. They may move around a lot, or even go the extra mile by running many miles a day or working out in the gym for hours. For these girls, moving is the way to maintain their skinny status. But just because a skinny girl is moving around a lot, doesn't mean she is now also eating a lot. In fact, many skinny girls who enjoy activities like running, often also don't overeat. One reason is that it can be difficult to maintain the level of energy they need for their workouts when eating too much food.

In college, before buying my first car, I used to walk around my college campus. Sometimes I would walk to a nearby restaurant or store. I felt alive and energized by my walks. When I got my car, things changed. I no longer walked everywhere; I drove instead. I continued to walk around on campus, from class to class though, while other students would waste their gas and drive from class to class, instead of walking. Although I enjoyed the convenience of my car, I also knew that cutting out my walking altogether would change the dynamics of my body. I needed to keep some activity in my life in order to maintain my skinny figure. I would also find myself walking upstairs when the elevator took too long or when I knew that walking up the stairs would take me to my destination quicker.

Walking from place to place is good, easy exercise and can help you maintain muscle mass, which helps to burn fat more easily. As long as your destination is reasonably close, walking to that destination can be a form of quick exercise and doesn't involve hours spent on the treadmill or working out with weights in that smelly gym. When the weather is nice, it's also great to get some fresh air into your lungs and enjoy the sun on your face. Riding a bicycle, taking stairs instead of the elevator, and parking further away allow a person to walk, and are good habits to get into. Each step or extra bit of physical activity you can add into your day will help push you towards your skinny goals. So trash the old thought that only working out in a gym will provide the exercise you need and start thinking about incorporating other ways to bring activity into your life! Just remember that being active does not mean doing difficult, strenuous, or tiresome physical activities. You can improve your health just by walking.

Exercise for the health of it

When a woman exercises it is typically to achieve weight loss or, at the very least, to keep from gaining more weight. When a man works out, they primarily do so to gain muscle mass and to stay fit. However, for both sexes, exercise is really all about one thing: to help them look and feel better. Other benefits exercise can give are decreased stress levels, increased happiness, better sleep and the ability to live longer. That's right! Being more active is proven to help lengthen life expectancy! If you are inactive, it is not too late for you to change your mindset and get moving.

To get you even more motivated to start moving, here is another fact: some leading causes of death are caused by a lack of physical activity. Believe it or not, non-activity plays a huge part in the deaths of millions of people. When you don't exercise and have little to no physical activity in your life, your muscles, joints and internal organs can start to atrophy. Have you ever had a long-term illness or a broken bone when you were unable to move around a lot? What happened once you were able to move around again? You were tired, your muscles were weak and your body had a hard time keeping up, right? That's because you were inactive. Over time, as you began incorporating more activity again into your life, you have more energy and are able to fend off diseases more easily.

Now consider if you never got up and moved around again for the rest of your life. Do you think your body would have the energy and stamina to keep all your body parts moving well into your later years? Probably not. Think about an elderly person stuck in a nursing home. They have only so much activity they can participate in and some are confined to their beds. Eventually their bodies shut down due to the lack of physical activity in their lives—their bodies simply do not have the stamina to keep up. Physical activity helps to keep the body functioning properly by providing muscle and energy to keep you going.

Exercises to get you moving

When some people think of exercising, they immediately think of expensive exercise equipment, gym memberships and personal trainers. They think that exercising will be expensive to perform, when in reality you can exercise without the use of equipment or with very little equipment. As I pointed out earlier, some of my exercise has come in the form of a simple walk. You don't need expensive gym memberships or high-priced equipment to get moving. Being a skinny girl is all about the mindset really—picking your eating plan and incorporating exercise that works best for you.

Some of the best exercises for losing weight are cardio exercises. Cardio exercising increases your heart rate, so you burn more calories. These types of exercises help improve the function of some of the organs in the body. Cardio can also help improve strength and enhance muscle and joint functioning. Once again, some people equate the word "cardio" with a negative connotation, but you can find the right kind of cardio for you. Do you love to dance? Dancing can be a terrific form of cardio and increases your blood flow, heart rate and builds stamina. What about biking? Get out the ol' Schwinn and take it for a twirl around the block! Get your kids or significant other involved too for a fun activity the whole family can enjoy. Plus, you'll see parts of your neighborhood you've probably never seen before all while getting a little of that dreaded cardio.

Another well-known cardio exercise is running. The best thing about running is that it does not require any equipment (except maybe a good pair of sneakers) which makes it one of the cheapest exercises. And you can find fun races of varying lengths in almost every town in the country. There are 5K's, 10K's, half marathons and whole marathons (for the most serious runner!) In addition, there are now fun runs; which usually involve short distances and are good for the whole family; mud runs, where competitors run through a variety of fun (and often muddy!) obstacle courses; and even trail running, which involves running through forests and over trails. There truly is something for everyone. Participating in an organized run helps some people to make goals for themselves as well as compare themselves to other runners. But remember: you are your own person and running (literally) your own race!

Don’t get bogged down with running statistics and times—it’s really about getting out there and having fun!

If running in competitions isn’t for you—here’s some great news! You can run almost anywhere. You can use a treadmill, you can run around a park or neighborhood or you can simply run in place—right in your own living room! And no one needs to know your time, your running abilities or that you stopped midway and walked the rest of the way! Remember that if you choose to run as an exercise, it doesn’t require you to run fast like people do in the Olympics and you don’t want to overdo it which may lead to injuries like shin splints, twisted ankles and runner’s knee. Every person will have their own speed and differences, according to their personal health and abilities, and you need to find that “sweet spot” for you. This will not only help to make the most of your workout, but will also help you to enjoy the exercise more so you will continue to make it part of a healthy routine.

Regardless of all the meanings and reasons people have for running, whether it is for fun, racing, or just to get healthy, it still gives the same benefits to your body. Running can decrease your risks of developing heart disease and strokes as well as increase muscle mass in your legs. Running has some psychological benefits too, like helping with depression. With so many great ways to run and with so many benefits—why NOT start running?

Another easy, basic exercise is walking. Walking is the most popular exercise and the most widely used by Americans. Almost everybody walks short distances to get to one place or another. Think about how much you walk in a given day. If you live in a two story home, you walk up and down stairs probably several times a day. If you live in a small town or even in a big city, you probably walk down to the local grocery or convenience store to pick up a few items instead of getting your car out of the garage. However, walking is not talked about as much as other exercises are, even though it is one of the safest exercises to perform and just about anyone can do it. Like running, walking requires no additional equipment except a good pair of shoes and you can walk just about anywhere. As a matter of fact, walking was one of the main ways of getting about in earlier times, before cars, trains and other modes of transportation were available. Imagine walking everywhere you had to go! What great exercise that must have been for your ancestors!

If you do choose walking as one of the exercises you want to try, there is one main thing you should keep in mind: walk with a buddy. It is best to find a walking buddy or group to enjoy your walks. Not only will it keep you company and pass the time as well, it will also make the walk more enjoyable when you have conversations with friends. Walking with a companion can also keep potential people from taking advantage of you, especially if you are in a large city. Walking alone, especially for a skinny girl, can be a dangerous activity. If you must walk alone, make sure you are aware of your surroundings at all times and avoid listening to music, which can impede your hearing and keep you from being mindful of your surroundings. Walking with friends or in a group will detract unsavory characters from bothering you and help to keep your walk safe and enjoyable.

As with many exercises, walking has its benefits. Walking, like running, improves your overall health and physical fitness by utilizing multiple parts of your body. Your legs will become stronger, your arms will be more toned and your overall posture will improve. We use walking for getting around the house, getting to our cars, and doing other day-to-day routines. However, you don't have to just walk in that simple way. To get the real benefits from walking, you need to go for longer distances, or walk shorter distances at a fast pace. If you choose to walk, make sure you wear good walking shoes that are comfortable and flexible, to prevent you from developing foot problems.

Another good exercise is bicycling. Bicycling can be done in different forms, such as riding to various places around your neighborhood, city or park and even on trails. An indoor exercise bicycle is a great way to start biking and it may be more comfortable especially in cities where rain and cold are more prevalent. Be sure to pick the right bike for your size and height. A good, comfortable seat is also important—if your seat isn't comfortable—you will NOT want to keep biking! Once you get biking around your neighborhood and become more comfortable on your bike, you'll find that your rides become longer and longer because you want to start exploring more and more places. Biking helps to increase your stamina, as well as your leg strength, and is a great way to start exploring!

Swimming is another way of exercising. Getting involved with sports is a way of exercising. Finding a job that requires a lot of moving around can be a form of exercise. Taking up dance lessons or any activity that involves movement can be a form of exercise. Also visiting a gym or joining a gym is a great idea. Whichever way you choose to exercise, you should find fun ways to incorporate exercise through various activities you do in your daily life.

Find something that will be fun and encouraging for you. When you begin your exercise program you might want to start it off with something simple and easy, then progress to more strenuous or complex exercises. If you want, you may seek the help of a personal fitness trainer to help you in losing weight and to help you learn more of the various exercises that can help. This can be expensive and demanding, but it can also be well worth the investment if you're unsure where to start or need a little motivation to get moving. But be sure to do research on which personal trainer would be best for you and don't be afraid to stop seeing them if it's not working out. In the end, it's about finding what's best overall for you and what fits into your schedule.

Break out of the ordinary

Exercising is unfortunately not everyone's cup of tea. Conventional weight loss methods like running, going to the gym, swimming or even playing a racquet sport may be boring for some people. Fortunately, there are hosts of new and unusual workout ideas that are so fun that it doesn't even feel like you're working out! Here are some of the more unusual workouts that you can try out today.

Zumba - This is the mother of all dance routines. This Latin-inspired dance fitness program combines elements of hip-hop, salsa, samba, Bollywood, belly dance, merengue, martial arts, squats and lunges to give you the workout of your life. Dances typically alternate between fast and slow tempos which helps burn an incredible amount of calories (between 500-1000 calories are burnt in a single session of Zumba!) Can't dance you say? No worries! Just keep moving along to the beat the best way you can—it's all about the activity anyway—not your rhythm!

AntiGravity® Yoga - We all know Yoga is an excellent, but rather slow, way of losing weight. Aerial Artist Christopher Harrison is the mastermind behind AntiGravity® Yoga, that combines all the good qualities of Yoga, Pilates, aerial acrobatics and calisthenics to create a workout that revolves around a hammock type apparatus. A challenging regime, it helps lose weight and tone up quickly. The basic principle is to merge athletic power with the creativity of dance. Although this may be a more challenging exercise, breaking out of your "working out is boring" comfort zone may be just the thing you need to jumpstart your exercise regime.

Piloxing - As the name so subtly suggests, this workout, created by former Ballerina Viveca Jensen, is a combination of boxing, dance and standing Pilates, creating a fat-burning, fun and fast-paced workout sure to get your whole body in shape and in tune. Piloxing combines cardiovascular workouts with flexibility for maximum calorie burning. Gloves with weights are worn as well while working out so that arms are sculpted, and fat burning occurs, during the process.

Spinning with Karaoke – Do you sing along with the tunes on your iPod while running or doing other exercising? Then this might be the class for you! While dance class workouts are in abundance, this one adds a unique twist to working out: Karaoke. The karaoke spin class combines a tough regime of cycling coupled with singing to your favorite tunes. Singing while cycling helps to keep track of your breathing as well as expand your lung capacity and stamina. If you can sing along without huffing and puffing, it means your body is prepared to train harder. This is a hot trend in America right now because it combines fun, functionality, and aids fitness enthusiasts (and amateur singers!) with losing weight fast.

That darn BMI again and how to get started

When you start incorporating more exercise into your life, you'll want to start tracking some things, including weight loss. Throughout your weight loss program, it is always best to keep track of how much weight you are losing, at the very least once a week. This is a good way to keep track of your goals and find out how close you are to meeting them. Before starting your weight loss program it's best to first determine your BMI. As I stated in the first chapter, your BMI is one of the ways that can indicate whether you are underweight, normal weight, overweight, or obese. This is a good starting point for your weight loss goals and can help you determine how much you need to lose. Figuring out your BMI is a simple calculation you can do by dividing how many pounds you weigh by how tall you are, squared. Example: BMI = (Weight in Pounds / (Height in inches x Height in inches) Then multiply that answer by 703. For example, let's say a person weighs 140 pounds and is 5'4" tall, which equals a total of 64 inches. Take 64 inches squared (64^2 or 64 x 64) and divide the number of pounds you weigh by 4096 (which is the result of 64 inches squared).

Next you want to take that number and multiply it by 703. Your final number should be similar to this number: 24.0283203125. You can round this number off to 24.03, making 24.03 your body mass index.

Here is what it would look like as a math equation:

BMI = 140 / 4096 x 703 = 24.03

If you're like me—math makes your brain hurt. Here's some good news: There are charts available online to save you the trouble and confusion of self-calculations if you find them to be too confusing.

Here is a simple chart to help you understand the categories of the BMI scale and to help you determine a starting point for your exercise and eating routine.

Category	**BMI Range – kg/m^2**
Severely Underweight	Less than 16.0
Underweight	From 16.0 to 18.5
Normal	From 18.5 to 25

Overweight	From 25 to 30
Obese Class I	From 30 to 35
Obese Class II	From 35 to 40
Obese Class III	Over 40

Keep in mind, like we said in Chapter 1, that this is only a starting point and should not be relied upon too heavily. Some people, like you after you start exercising, may weigh more as they gain muscle mass. The BMI scale is a "general" outlook on your overall health and is to be used as a starting place for your routine only. As you progress, you will factor in your weight, your overall health and your stamina as additional points to consider on your journey.

So many people start their exercise regime at a pace that they cannot sustain and this causes them to give up quickly. When beginning any exercise program of your own, it is best to start out at a slower pace, especially if it is your first time. Starting out slower will prevent you from overstressing yourself and from becoming too tired, too quickly and, eventually, giving up. You want to gradually increase how many exercises you do, or increase the amount of time you spend exercising. As your body becomes more acclimated with daily exercise, you can increase the length of your routine or increase weights you may be using. Never push your body too far too quickly—be consistent and persistent as you move forward. Put it this way: If you go full speed and push yourself today to your utmost limits…you probably won't be able to walk tomorrow, much less do any exercise. Push yourself, but know your limits. That way you can do it again tomorrow—creating an ongoing regime for your ultimate fitness goals. The very first thing anyone should do when beginning a workout is to stretch and warm-up. Warm-up exercises, like light jogging in place or simple jumping jacks, are the exercises you perform before doing more strenuous exercises to help your body prepare and perform better. These do just what the names suggest: they warm up your body for the more strenuous exercises to come. This helps you to avoid injury as well as sends the signal to your body: Hey! We're going to exercise now!

Getting the most for your body

One of those most dreaded physical attributes for just about anyone is the dreaded belly paunch. Stomach fat is not only unsightly, but is also considered one of the fats you should rid from your body. Belly fat puts you at a higher risk for developing heart diseases and other illnesses such as type-two diabetes. In younger women, body fat tends to be focused in the buttocks, hips and thighs areas. But older women see body fat shifting to the dreaded belly area. As people age, muscle fat tends to account for a lot of our body weight, while muscle mass decreases. Decreased muscle mass makes it harder to lose weight, but muscles are used in your body to burn off added fats (which causes our weight issues). As women age, especially during the menopausal years, their estrogen levels decrease. This often causes an increase in belly fat too. This is why it is so important, especially for young women (even if they think they have great metabolism or are "naturally thin"), to get moving now before their bodies start changing and adding more and more fat.

In older women, this lack of estrogen causes the fat to shift to the belly area. You don't necessarily have to gain weight for fat to shift. According to WebMD, "Belly fat has been linked to an increased risk of heart disease and diabetes" and they "found that people with the most belly fat had about double the risk of dying prematurely as people with the least amount of belly fat." But the good news is there are wonderful exercises that can help you to combat these issues as well as look your best.

As discussed, exercises, such as walking and jogging, can help you to lose body fat and your typical sit-ups or crunches are a great way to convert the belly fat to muscle mass in your stomach area. Belly fat is just one of the many areas you should be concerned about during your new exercise routine. Legs, arms, buttocks, thighs and even your back muscles are important areas to focus on. It's important to make sure you're doing exercises that can help with every area of your body to help ensure you are getting the best total workout.

Here are some great exercises for different areas of your body:

Legs, thighs, buttocks	Squats, lunges, stair climbing, biking, running
Arms, back	Swimming, weights, running, push-ups
Stomach	Sit-ups, planks, running

Try to pick a variety of workouts for every body part as well as your overall physique. This will not only ensure that you are targeting each and every part, but also to keep you from becoming bored with your workout.

Once again, we see that it's not about just one or two things, it's about the overall package of what needs to happen to be a skinny girl. But, once again, it's not about torturing yourself, but it's about finding what works right for you both for fun and health.

CHAPTER THREE: THE TRUTH ABOUT EATING LIKE A SKINNY GIRL (RECIPES INCLUDED!)

What is the largest skinny girl food myth? That skinny girls don't like to eat! Skinny girls not only like to eat, but they have learned how to eat good food (or when to stop eating) to help maintain their skinny girl status. In this chapter, we'll discuss the right foods to choose and even share some simple recipes that you can start using today!

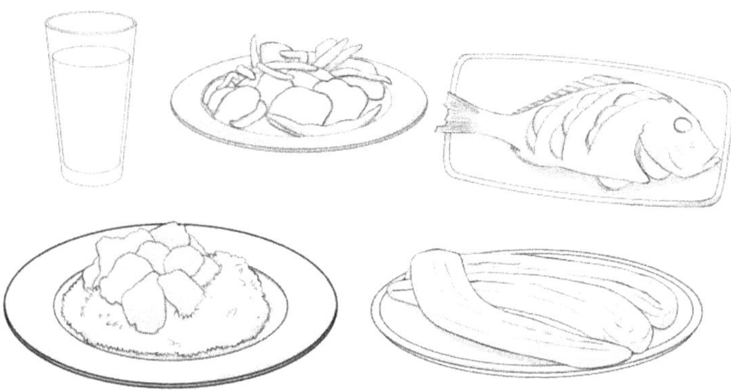

There are so many diet foods labeled "all natural," "low fat," "gluten free," "organic" and so many others out on the market today that it's hard to know what are our best options. We're inundated with what this "expert"

recommends, what our friends tell us works for them and our own stubborn ways of eating so we just keep making bad choices! But I'm here to tell you that it's easier than it seems. Let's look at some simple food options, their benefits and even some fun recipes to get us started on the right path!

Burble, Cluck and Moo

Meat is the primary food staple for most people (except vegetarians and vegans). Some of the healthiest meats are fish (burble), poultry (cluck) and grass-fed beef (moo) (there is also lamb and buffalo).

There is a lot of debate about "grass fed" versus "organic," so let's discuss the differences. Grass fed means that the animal was allowed to forage and graze for their own fresh, natural food. Although they may be given substitutes in the winter months, the goal is to provide them with the most natural food possible. Non-grass fed animals are mainly fed foods that they wouldn't eat naturally, such as grains and soybeans. Eating these foods changes the animal's composition of fat in their bodies. For example, a farm-raised animal that mainly eats grain or corn has higher omega-6 fatty acids and lower omega-3 fatty acid levels.

Omega-3 fatty acids and omega-6 fatty acids are polyunsaturated fats that are essential for the human body. Omega-3 fatty acids and omega-6 fatty acids are consumed through foods and are not produced in the body. These are beneficial to the human body. These foods are also higher in calories and provide a larger end-product (i.e. fatter cow = bigger steak / bigger YOU).

The benefits of eating omega-3 fatty acids are a decreased risk of heart disease and cancer. It can boost brainpower, reduce the risk of becoming obese, and reduce the risk of blood clotting. Omega-3 fatty acids also improve the immune system. You can find omega-3 fatty acids in fish, olive oil, nuts, beans and grass-fed cattle. You can also find them in red meat, vegetable oil and dairy products. Your body needs these fatty acids to help improve its functioning, but eating too many omega-6 fatty acids is unhealthy, so they should be consumed in moderation. Organic deals more with how the animal is raised. They cannot be confined in feedlots, placed in unsanitary conditions and cannot be exposed to artificial pesticides, fertilizers, antibiotics (for prolonged periods), GMOs, hormones or other synthetic contaminants. This often includes being grass fed and creates an overall healthier animal.

Both are actually wonderful, healthy eating options, but it's difficult to know for sure what you're getting unless you see the farm the animal has come from.

In addition to learning where your meat comes from, there are also different methods you can use when cooking meat. As you may know, frying or deep-frying food is not a healthy way to cook food, because it drains foods of their essential nutrients and adds fat. Especially if you are eating non-grass fed animals, you should stray from frying as it only adds more fat to your already fatty meat.

Some of the healthier methods are baking, broiling, pressure-cooking and grilling. Here are a few simple recipes to help get you started eating healthier.

Baked Fish (4 servings)

Ingredients:

- 1 – 1.5 lb. fish of your choice (Tilapia, Cod and Haddock work well)
- 4 Tbl. melted butter or olive oil
- Additional seasonings to taste

Preheat oven to 425 degrees Fahrenheit. If your fish is not already scaled and cleaned, you want to make sure you get that done quickly. If you're unsure how to do this—check with your local butcher. The next step is to pat the fish dry with a clean paper towel and place it in a lightly greased 9" x 13" glass-baking pan. Brush both sides of the fish gently with the butter or olive oil. Season both sides of the fish with your choice of seasonings. (Dill, salt, black pepper, lemon pepper, paprika, and Old Bay are all good seasoning options for fish.) Bake for twenty to thirty minutes. When the fish is opaque and flakes lightly – it is done.

Nutritional info per serving: Approx. 200 calories (depending on the fish used), 14 grams of fat and 24 grams of protein.

Grilled Chicken (4 servings)

- *Ingredients:*
  2 to 3 pounds of chicken parts (legs, thighs) – skin removed
- 4 Tbl. melted butter or olive oil
- Salt and pepper to taste
- Additional seasonings to taste

Preheat grill to about 400 degrees Fahrenheit. Brush melted butter or olive oil on chicken. Sprinkle the chicken parts with salt, black pepper and seasonings of your choice. Typical seasonings used are paprika, garlic powder and onion powder (but experiment with seasonings you prefer!) Place the chicken on the grill and close lid. Grill for 4 to 6 minutes per side. The cooking time will vary depending on what type of grill and the parts of the chicken you are using. Chicken should be cooked to at least 165 degrees internal temperature. You can check this with a cooking thermometer.

Nutritional info per serving: Approx. 135 calories (depending on chicken parts used), 13 grams of fat and 5 grams of protein.

Green leafy goodness and sweet fruity options

Everyone knows that fruits and vegetables are important to our health. They provide our bodies with much needed vitamins, minerals and fiber as well as help prevent us from developing chronic diseases. Not everyone likes fruits and vegetables, but consuming a balanced amount of these important foods can prevent you from developing heart disease, stroke and cancers.

Vitamins and minerals are essential for helping our body grow properly. Without vitamins and minerals, bones can deteriorate and become brittle, growth can be stunted and our overall health can be compromised.

Fiber helps to lessen the risk of diabetes, heart disease, constipation and even assists with weight loss. It also slows the movement of foods in the intestines, which in turn, eases hunger and food intake. Soluble fibers swell, causing you to believe you are full, decreasing your desire of overeating.

Many people don't eat as much fruits and vegetables as they should mostly because many don't like the taste of vegetables, and some say they would rather eat foods that taste better than veggies. Let's be honest, a donut tastes better than kale. But a lifetime of donuts will not help us to maintain our weight or feel healthy. When you're craving that sweetness, opt for a sweet fruit instead. At least you'll get the fiber benefits and your sweet tooth will be satisfied. It's not about torturing ourselves—it's about finding foods we enjoy AND are good for us. In my opinion, fruits are one of the healthiest desserts a person can eat and there are many options to get that sweet fix. In addition, fruits and vegetables are convenient to eat. There isn't much prep work needed—most just need washed off or peeled. Look at some of these recipes and see how easy it is to include fruits and vegetables in your life.

Fruit Salad (4 servings)

Ingredients:

- 2 peeled, seeded mandarin oranges, cut into bite-sized chunks or use 1 cup of canned mandarin oranges (be sure to drain off the syrup if included)
- 1 Tbl. lemon juice
- 1/3 cup honey
- 2 large apples or 1 large pear, cut into bite-sized chunks
- 1 cup peaches or nectarines, cut into bite-sized chunks
- 1 cup seedless grapes, cut in half
- Combine all ingredients together. Serve chilled. (That was easy, right?)

Nutritional info per serving: Approx. 153 calories, less than 1 gram of fat and 2.5 grams of dietary fiber. In addition, this recipe provides 5% of your daily Vitamin A, and 13% of your Vitamin C – a healthy dose of vitamins for your day!

Baked Bananas (4 servings)

Ingredients:

- 4 medium bananas in their skins
- Lemon juice
- Honey, brown sugar, or Confectioner's sugar (optional)

Preheat your oven to 375 degrees Fahrenheit. Place the four bananas in a baking dish. Bake the bananas for about 20 minutes or until their skins turn black and start to split. Serve the bananas hot in their skins. Open the bananas, sprinkle them with lemon juice and either honey, brown sugar or confectioner's sugar.

Nutritional info per serving: Approx. 121 calories, less than 1 gram of fat and 3 grams of dietary fiber. In addition, this provides 34% of your daily Vitamin B-6!

Green Beans and Potatoes (4 servings)

Ingredients:

- 1 lb. trimmed green beans
- 4 medium boiling potatoes, peeled and halved
- 1 onion, chopped (optional)
- Salt and pepper to taste
- Other seasonings to taste (Bay Leaf is a good option) (optional)

Place enough water in a medium-sized pot to cover the green beans and potatoes and bring to a boil. Add the pound of green beans and potatoes, as well as the onion, if desired. Then simmer the pot while covered for about 15 minutes or until beans are tender. Drain and season to taste.

Nutritional info per serving: Approx. 191 calories, less than 1 gram of fat and 9 grams of dietary fiber. In addition, this dish is full of potassium, Vitamin A, Vitamin B-6, and Vitamin C.

Baked Eggplant (2 servings)

Ingredients:

- 2 medium eggplants, 1 lb. each
- Olive oil, vegetable oil, or melted/softened butter
- Seasonings, as desired

Wipe the outside of the eggplant, then peel the eggplant and cut into half-inch thick slices. Soak pieces in salt water overnight in the fridge. Using salt will help draw the water out of the eggplant and help it to be less mushy. The following day, drain eggplant and rinse with water. Preheat the oven to 400 degrees Fahrenheit. Brush the slices on both sides with oil or butter and season to taste. Place pieces on a baking sheet and bake for about 15-20 minutes or until tender, turning the eggplants once during baking.

Nutritional info per serving: Approx. 129 calories, 7 grams of fat and 5 grams of dietary fiber. (Nutritional value will vary depending on how much oil/butter and what seasonings are used.)

Dairy products

Dairy products are milk or products made from milk, such as cheese, butter and yogurt. Dairy foods are good sources of Vitamin D and calcium. We mostly consume our milk from animals, like cows and goats. There are additional "dairy" products on the market now in the form of almond milk, soymilks and other plant based dairy products. If you are lactose intolerant, these may be great options for you, but check into each to determine which has the best nutritional value.

Dairy foods are great for developing strong and healthy bones and can significantly reduce the risk of osteoporosis, a disease of the bones that decreases bone density and tissue. This disease is more common in women than men, particularly older women.

One glass of whole milk has 150 calories and 5 grams of fat, but 8 grams of protein and also gives you 30% of your daily calcium requirement. Cheese is another good source of protein and calcium, but be careful adding too much to your diet as it is also high in fat. There are a variety of cheeses in the world—sample and experiment with which ones you prefer.

The Dreaded Carb!

Foods in the grain group come from different plants such as rye, rice, wheat and oats. These foods include bread, cereal and noodles. The grain group also provides our bodies with carbohydrates which makes glucose—a fuel that provides energy to our bodies. Carbohydrates have been given a bad rap in the past few years due to the glucose (or sugar) issue. Some people feel that carbs can make us fat, but adding in the right carbohydrates to your diet can actually help you stay thin. Look for carbs with higher dietary fiber and without white flour and added sugars. “Good” carbs are defined as foods that have more fiber and complex carbohydrates and that break down though digestion before your body can use it as a glucose source.

Often, many of us eat grains that have been refined and exhausted of their nutrients. An example of this is white bread, which uses white flour. Opt for whole grain wheat bread instead, which is more easily digestible by your body. Cutting out all carbs from your diet will only make you sluggish and have less energy. Choose whole grain options and keep the dreaded carb!

Like I’ve mentioned earlier, picking up a sweet snack is sometimes easier than figuring out what is the best option to choose. Here are some ideas to get you started making healthier decisions: Eat brown rice instead of white. Use long grain brown rice instead of the five minute instant. Try flax seed breads or even flax seeds sprinkled on your cereal. Crackers come in whole grain too. In fact, if you look carefully, your grocery store is FILLED with whole grain options now.

But be sure to check that label—look for higher dietary fiber and lower sugar options. When choosing whole grain products, if possible, make sure the first ingredient is whole grains or whole grain flour, not enriched white flour.

Indian Rice Curry (6 servings)

Ingredients:

- 3 Tbl. olive oil
- 1 small onion, diced
- 1/4 cup chopped apple (Tart is nice)
- 2 tsps. Curry powder
- Dash of cayenne pepper (optional)
- 4 cups of cooked brown rice (cook in low sodium chicken/vegetable stock for extra flavor)
- 2 cups canned chickpeas, drained
- 1 Tbl. lemon juice
- Black Pepper (to taste)

In a heavy skillet pan, sauté the onions in olive oil for about three minutes. Add the apple and sauté for another three minutes. Add the curry and cayenne powder if desired. Then coat the onion and apples, adding cooked rice and chickpeas. As soon as the dish is hot all the way through, add pepper to taste. Sprinkle it with lemon juice and serve.

Nutritional info per serving: 315 calories, 9 grams of fat and 7 grams of dietary fiber.

I hope this chapter has given you some good information, dispelled a few food myths and helped you start choosing good options for your daily eating. Being a skinny girl isn't about not eating—it's about eating right!

CHAPTER FOUR: MY FOOD HAS WHAT IN IT?

Do you really know what you are putting into your body? Frank talk will scare you skinny in no time, but we're here to shine a light on the good, the bad and the ugly within your food. In this chapter we'll discuss trans fats, salt, sugars, pesticides, preservatives and the REAL scoop on "diet" foods.

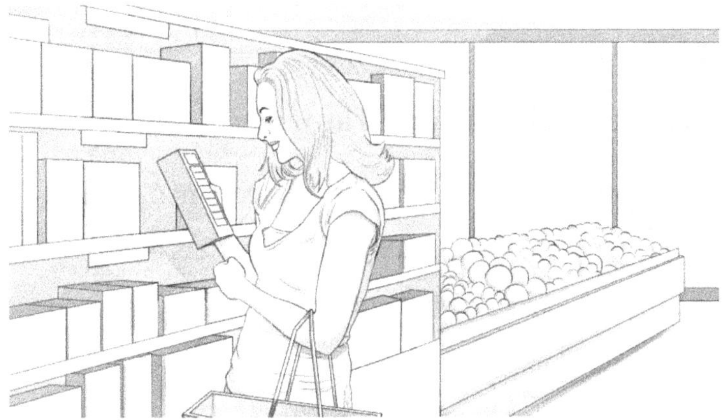

Food makes the world go round, but what we eat in one country, does not always translate to what other people eat in their countries, or even in different areas of our own country. For example, people who live in coastal areas have access to fresh seafood like fish, scallops, shrimp and even lobster. But it's harder for someone in Middle America, like Nebraska, to get fresh seafood on a regular basis. They rely more heavily on corn products instead. Likewise, a dairy farmer may rely more on beef and milk products, but a native person living in the wild may have diets full of products from the land—like plants. Certainly, these differences have some bearing on the health and weight of each individual.

Fat, Sugar and Sodium – The Basics

The word "trans fats" has become a common part of our vocabulary, but really what is it? Trans fats are uncommon in nature, but are commercially produced from vegetable fat for margarine, packaged baked goods, and snack foods. Whenever you look at a food package to see if it contains trans fats, check for its other name: "partially-hydrogenated oils." Trans fats are unhealthy and pose many risks. Trans fats are used in deep fryers in a lot of fast food restaurants and are used because they last longer and can be reused over again many times. (Think about *that* the next time you buy something deep-fried.) Trans fats are also cheap and enhance the flavor of many foods. (That's why we love fast food and fried food so much!)

Although trans fats are certainly edible, millions of people ingest them every day, they have been consistently linked with coronary heart disease. These types of fats are known for increasing LDL cholesterol, also known as the bad cholesterol, and decreasing HDL cholesterol, which is known as the good kind. LDL cholesterol contributes to a thick, hard deposit that can clog arteries and make them less flexible. This means a clot can form and narrow your arteries potentially causing a stroke or heart attack. HDL cholesterol helps remove LDL from the arteries and may protect against things like stroke and heart disease. Obviously, it's better to have more HDL than LDL.

Trans fats can also increase the risk of health problems such as obesity, cancer, diabetes and liver failure. But this doesn't seem to faze most people. In fact, although consumption of trans fats have decreased in recent years, according to the Centers for Disease Control and Prevention, Americans still ingest approximately 1.3 grams of artificial trans fat each day.

In America, fast food restaurants seem to inundate every corner and our lives are increasingly too busy for sit-down family meals made by Mom. Instead, Americans frequent the convenient restaurants that dot the landscape, filling their diets with nothing but these unhealthy trans fats. Unfortunately, if a person does not balance out these unhealthy meals with healthier ones, made from natural fruits and vegetables, their life span may be shorter than they realize.

These fast food restaurants are interested in making money. They utilize these unhealthy cooking oils because it's cheap, works well and helps their bottom line. But, with the emergence of more nutritional guidelines, requirements from the government, and backlash from their consumers, these same restaurants have now begun to implement and serve healthier options. In fact, now that trans fats have been determined to be such a risk to our health, food labels and packaging also are required to list the amount of trans fat in products. It's a trend in the right direction.

Keep in mind: no one is forcing you to eat these foods. There are other alternatives, and there is no one stopping you from eating healthier. It is not the restaurants duty to make sure you eat well—it's your health and you need to make the decisions.

There is a type of trans fat present in the milk and body fat of some mammals in small quantities such as cattle and sheep. However, artificial trans fats are consumed today way more than those naturally occurring ones. The *American Heart Association* recommends limiting your trans fat intake to less than one percent of your total daily calories (remember the statistic earlier – most people have over 1.3 grams a day which is roughly 4% or more of your daily intake). Your diet needs some fats in it, but you should be aware of what kind of fats you are ingesting and what the recommended daily amount is, so you can avoid going over your daily-recommended amount.

Use this chart as a way to figure out your daily intake:

0 g (trans fat) / 0.5 g (total fat) x 100 = 0% from trans fat

The healthier alternatives to trans fats are monounsaturated fats, which can be found naturally in peanuts, canola oils, avocados and olives. These fats reduce the amount of LDL cholesterol (the bad kind, remember?) from your body. Mediterranean countries tend to eat more fat in their diets, but it is rich in these monounsaturated fats (olives, nuts, fish, lamb), not the trans fats we are so used to here in America.

Restaurants and food manufacturers use more than tasty trans fats to entice their customers, they are also using chemicals and artificial coloring to attract consumers. And these artificial colors and chemicals also can be harmful to our health. For instance, how often have you made macaroni and cheese from a box? Do you think that cheese naturally comes in that color? Check the box. Do you see "artificial color" or FD&C

Red No. 40? That means they have used artificial means to color your yummy mac and cheese. In the U.K. these types of food are required to have a warning label attached (due to potential harm it may cause to children), but not here in the U.S. That's why it's important to be diligent and educated about what we put into our bodies every day.

In addition, there is a lot of sodium, or salt in the foods we eat as well. Eating too much salt can raise blood pressure to an unhealthy level, which can lead to a plethora of other health risks. But the salt in our diets comes from more than the salt shaker on the table. Once again, fast foods and packaged foods contain the bulk of our sodium consumption. If you are trying to reduce the amounts of sodium in your body, try to buy fresh foods instead and check the amount of sodium listed on the label of any packaged foods. The recommended amount of sodium is less than 2400 mg per day.

However, some sodium in our diets is healthy. Sodium can help to balance fluids in the body and help muscles to relax. It can also help nerves run smoothly and organs function properly. Once again, it's important to be diligent about what we're putting in our bodies. It's up to us to keep track and know what's healthy.

Another product that is present in most foods we eat is sugar. There has been much debate about white-granulated sugar versus high-fructose corn syrup, but sugar is sugar and it should be limited in our diets no matter what, if you want to maintain that skinny girl figure. However, it's important once again to check the labels of any foods you're consuming. If the ingredient list mainly consists of sugar or sugar based products—stay away! Steer clear from products containing any combination of these words in the label: corn sweetener, corn syrup, sugar, dextrose, glucose, honey, maltose, sucrose, treacle, xyclose and maple sugar. (There are more—this is only a partial list!) You might be surprised what foods you find these products in—it isn't just desserts and sweets. Soft drinks, jams and preserves, cereals and even dried fruits have a lot of added sugars so be sure to check your labels!

Like many other foods we've discussed, sugar should only be eaten in moderation, as too much of it can cause health problems and weight gain. Sugar can also slow your immune system, promote tooth decay, and cause liver damage. Hypoglycemia, osteoporosis and cardiovascular disease may also result from eating too much sugar. The majority of these above-mentioned products: sugar, sodium and fats; are generally found in unhealthy foods. Fast foods, pre-packaged foods and many of the other delicious things we love to eat contain too much of these potentially health altering products. Eating these products in moderation, checking food labels each and every time and adding more natural foods to our diet is a good first step.

Pesticides

Did you know that some farm-raised fruits and vegetables can contain pesticides?

Pesticides are chemicals or substances that farmers use to destroy and keep away pests such as insects, animals, bacteria and fungi. Many people use pesticides in their own homes to kill spiders, wasps and ants. Farmers use pesticides mainly in an effort to keep pests from destroying or spoiling crops. Although pesticides can be very helpful in keeping plants from becoming destroyed and can also enable the farmers to produce more fruits and vegetables, they can also be harmful to consumers and pose many health risks.

Pesticides have been linked to everything from headaches and nerve damage, to skin irritations and even cancer. Children, the elderly and those with pre-existing health conditions are more vulnerable to pesticides, which can cause cancers, nerve damage, immune system disorders and birth defects in children. It has been said that many people who deal with pesticides, such as farmers, have been poisoned by them. Recent studies indicate that pesticides, used in farm and country living, may also attribute to Parkinson's disease; a disease of the brain that affects nerve cells that control muscle movement in our bodies like walking. The disease is basically a disorder of the central nervous system that greatly affects one's motor skills causing difficulty in walking, muscle tremors and muscle response rate. Childhood leukemia has been linked to prenatal exposure of residential pesticides. Leukemia is a group of cancers that usually begins in the bone marrow and results in high numbers of abnormal white blood cells. These abnormal white blood cells are called leukemia cells. Leukemia cells inhibit normal blood cells from performing their roles in the body, and leukemia cells life spans are longer than needed.

There are alternatives to traditional pesticides, such as pesticide devices; biologically-based pesticides are safer than chemical pesticides. For smaller gardens, encouraging natural wildlife, such as bats and birds to roost and nest nearby can help with the bug population.

The FDA recommends washing your fruits and vegetables thoroughly before eating or even cutting them. Wash your hands before touching the produce and then wash the produce off with plain running water. Use your fingers to rub away any dirt on the outside and discard the outer leafs of vegetables like lettuce. Once washed, dry the produce with a clean, dry towel to get any additional dirt or pesticides off. Cutting off the outer skin helps reduce your risks and pulling off any bruised or discolored sections of the produce, as this may be a sign of contamination, is another smart move. Even though people generally wash off their produce, it can still affect our health. The best way to avoid pesticides on your fruits and vegetables would be to grow the produce yourself. But if that's not possible then choosing organic, which prohibits the use of most pesticides, is your best option.

Preservatives

You probably don't give much thought to the preservation of your food, but a majority of what we eat every day uses some type of preservative. Preservatives have been used for centuries in our food to keep it from spoiling, to prevent bacteria growth and to help it last longer. There are several ways we preserve our food including pickling, refrigeration, freezing, pasteurization, canning, dehydration and the use of chemical preservatives.

The positive effects of preserving are obvious, but there are some negative effects as well. Certain chemical preservatives can cause health problems such as respiratory problems. Food additives and preservatives have also been linked to developmental changes in young children, perhaps causing hyperactive behavior.

To avoid unneeded health issues, it's best to stick with foods that contain little to no preservatives. This means you'll need to eat it quickly or refrigerate it immediately. Buying and eating fresh is really the way to go.

Don't let this chapter scare you! The foods we eat are made up of more than what meets the eye, and sometimes people don't take the time to read up on their favorite foods. Trans fats and pesticides can leave residue in and on the foods we consume, but are still safe to eat, in moderation. Be mindful of what you eat and what the food you're putting in your mouth contains. If the label contains a bunch of words you can't pronounce – it's probably best to put it back. As I mentioned before, eating organic or growing your own food is the best possible solution, but can also be more expensive and time-consuming in the end. You will have to decide what is your best option to eat healthier, be the skinny girl you want to be and to avoid health issues along the way.

EXTRA: "Low Fat" and Diet Pills Myths

When you go to the grocery store or supermarket today, you often find a whole section of foods labeled with one of these phrases, “low-fat, lite, light, sugar-free, fat-free, low-calorie” or simply “diet.” Naturally, for people who want to lose weight, these seem like the perfect food choices. They sell tremendously and are very popular with people who believe that if they eat low fat food, they’ll lose weight quickly and easily. After all, the manufacturers seem to be looking out for our health by pointing out which foods are “healthier,” right? However if you delve into the reality behind these terms you will be shocked to find out the real truth.

The FDA deems that any food with three grams or less of fat can be labeled as “low fat“ but this doesn’t take into account the sodium or calorie content. In fact, many manufacturers just decrease the serving size of their products to accommodate this rule. That means, it isn’t really lower in fat than it was last week – there is just less to eat! Breakfast bars are one example of a “diet“ food that is advertised as being healthy and nutritious, but some contain as much fat and sugar as a regular piece of chocolate. (And who wouldn't rather have a piece of chocolate over a breakfast bar?) Remember to always read the entire nutritional label – not just the "diet" label on the front of the packaging. Pick items with fewer ingredients, and more vitamins and minerals.

People often confuse products that claim to have "no sugar" in them as good diet options too. As we discussed earlier in this chapter, sugar can lead to obesity and many health problems. Because of this, many people choose to avoid natural sugars all together and replace them with "sweeteners" and products that claim to have no "added" sugar. Unfortunately, these sweeteners can cause more health issues than just eating a smaller portion of real sugar and products that claim to have no sugar are probably lying (see earlier part of chapter).

It has been proposed by some health food professionals that many manufacturers and marketers simply use these "hot button" words to get you, the consumer, to purchase their products. As a consumer, we need to be educated and not let others dictate what we put into our bodies. In the end, they are our bodies and we need to treat them with the utmost care that we can. Reading this book is a good start at educating yourself to some of these myths and bad food manufacturer tactics. Remember to read every label and know what you're reading!

In addition to the "diet" food myth, there are a lot diet supplements and pills available over the counter today that entice you with promises of helping you lose weight quickly and easily with virtually no effort from your side. They promise to literally burn away your fat and melt the calories into oblivion.

If it was possible to burn away years of bad eating by just popping a few diet pills, why do people waste their time working out in the gym and avoiding their favorite foods? Furthermore, why are there "low fat" and "diet" food options! It's all a marketing scam – don't give in.

The worst part about some of these diet pills, and what makes them even more off limits, is that they're not just ineffective, some of them are potentially harmful. The reasons they are available over the counter without the FDA clamping down on them is because diet supplements and weight loss pills do not go through the strict tests and high standards applied to other prescription drugs. (Check and see – most of these products contain wording like "These statements not evaluated by the Food and Drug Administration." This means that they are not held to the safety guidelines put forth – they are just "claims" – not actual "proof.") The FDA eventually had diet supplements containing Phenylpropanolamine (a stroke causing ingredient) removed – unfortunately, *after* people suffered from strokes - but it brings to light how dangerous these supplements can be. People must suffer health consequences *before* the FDA can step in. Weight loss pills and supplements have been associated with causing cardiovascular problems as well as being responsible for a number of mysterious deaths.

Although “diet“ products and fat burning pills claim to be the miracle cure for weight loss, they are not as miraculous as we would want them to be.

The lesson we can take away from this is that getting skinny has no easy route, so it’s important to be diligent in reading labels, making good healthy food choices and don’t take short cuts!

CHAPTER FIVE: VEGETARANIANISM AND VEGANISM ARE NOT FOR EVERYONE

I'm sure you've been told that a good way to lose weight is to adapt a vegetarian or vegan diet. It certainly does work for some, but not for others. In this chapter, we'll delve into the do's and don'ts of these specific diets and help you decide if it's right for your skinny girl journey.

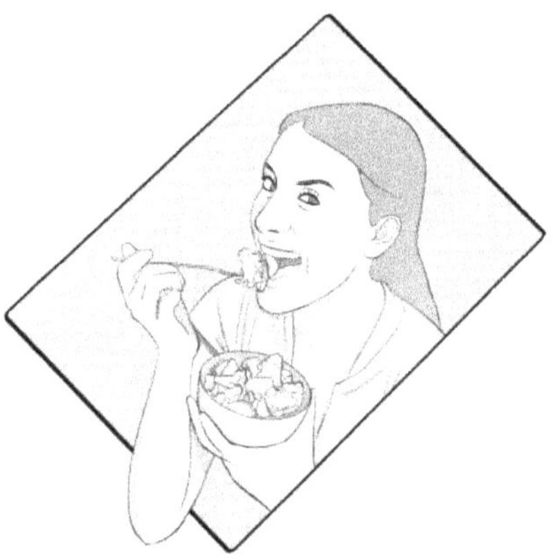

Vegetarianism is a dietary practice that focuses on the consumption of fruits and vegetables with the idea of abstaining from consumption of animal meat and animal based products. While some people adopt this diet for ethical, health, religious or cultural reasons there are aesthetic purposes to vegetarianism as well.

How Vegetarianism can help you get skinny

Many people view vegetarianism as a restrictive type of diet. But, according to some medical studies vegetarians, on average, eat approximately 500 calories less than non-vegetarians, which means they may have an easier time maintaining a skinny lifestyle. In fact, avid followers of the vegetarian diet believe that going vegetarian can aid you in losing weight even if you don't supplement it by a rigorous exercise regime. (Sounds better than diet pills, right?)

In addition, some research has proven that people who have grown up on vegetarian diets tend to be leaner than their meat-eating counterparts, helping to maintain their weight over time. The theory behind this is that fruits, vegetables, and protein-filled plants are filling and have a lower calorie count while a non-vegetarian diet likely has more saturated fat. (Being vegetarian keeps sounding better and better…)

Dr. Susan Berkow and Dr. Neal Barnard, both from the Physicians Committee for Responsible Medicine, conducted a weight study of vegetarians versus non-vegetarians. The study was conducted over short periods of time and participants were specifically told not to alter their workout habits so that the weight loss would be completely related to the food intake and no other factors. Their study showed that over half the people studied, who followed a vegetarian diet, weighed less than those on a meat-based diet.

Being vegetarian is also a good way to detoxify your body because you will consume larger amounts of vitamins, minerals and fiber rather than the toxic chemicals that certain types of fish and meat are known to contain. (And the preservatives we discussed in the last chapter.) As we discussed in previous chapters, eating your own grown fruits and vegetables is possibly the safest way to know what's going into your body. This is basically being vegetarian.

While the goal of this book is to give you advice on how to lose weight, be skinny and maintain your lower body weight, it is essential for me to give you tips that will help you achieve an overall healthiness. While we all desire to be skinny, I believe that being healthy is the first step in the skinny girl process.

Lettuce Tread Lightly

Based on the excellent advantages of going vegetarian as mentioned above, you might be swayed to quickly switch to this dietary choice in your bid to get skinny, but there are some important pointers to remember when it comes to being vegetarian. Switching to a vegetarian diet doesn't mean you will automatically lose weight. Once again, as I've stated before, you still need to make smart choices. There are plenty of "vegetarian" foods on the market (just like those "low fat" and "diet" options I mentioned in the last chapter.) All of these foods may or may not actually be a healthy alternative. Being vegetarian is not a "quick fix" or a "sure thing" when it comes to losing weight. You will still not lose weight if you eat large quantities of vegetarian food – you still need to consider calories!

Remember to stay away from white pasta, bread and rice and try to switch these with their whole grain versions. Even though potatoes are a staple of the vegetarian diet, they do lead to weight gain and can cause high cholesterol problems, so it is always better to have reduced amount of potatoes on your plate. Strive to maintain a healthy balance in all the foods you eat by having a starch, vegetable and protein in each meal. A lot of people have the misconception that eating fruits regularly is healthy and will help alleviate weight gain, but a lot of fruits are high in sugar, like apples, watermelon and mango. Although eating an apple is obviously better than eating a donut, remember to consider all your options – is there a better fruit option? YES! It is better to eat low calorie fruits like berries and citrus fruits if you want to lose weight. For vegetarians, dairy products are very important too, but ensure that you buy low calorie and reduced fat yogurts, milks and cheeses.

Vegetarian diets are fiber and protein rich, but it is only meat, chicken and fish that are rich in zinc and iron, which is highly essential for a healthy body. Be sure to educate yourself on what your body needs for proper nutrition and consult your doctor when switching to a new eating lifestyle. Vitamin supplements may be needed to maintain the proper balance.

Remember that a vegetarian diet by itself is not a weight loss plan. But following a healthy vegetarian diet by eating the right foods in the balanced proportions will help you lose more weight as compared to when you are on a non-vegetarian diet. You will probably find that you crave meat and other comfort foods when you first try to eat healthier as well. All human beings have "comfort" foods that they turn to and, for some people, this is the cause of their weight gain. Be patient and don't torture yourself! If you fall off the vegetarian wagon – just get back on the next time you eat. Eventually, your body will acclimate to your new way of eating.

Vegetarian Diet Goodies

If you are on a vegetarian diet and feel like you have over stretched the recipes that you have and are looking for something different, here are a few innovations that will spice up your diet.

Low-calorie Potato Chips

While we all enjoy gorging on potato chips, we're doing ourselves, and our goal to be healthy and thin, a disservice by eating the fried potato chips that we buy at the grocery store and at fast food restaurants. As we discussed in an earlier chapter, they use those trans fats that are so damaging for our systems. For a quick and easy potato fix that'll spice up your palate and keep you right on track on your weight loss goal, try this low-calorie potato chip recipe. It may seem childishly simple but its beauty is in its simplicity. You can switch up the taste too – just by using different spices!

Ingredients:

- Four Potatoes, unpeeled and scrubbed clean
- Olive Oil
- Salt & Pepper
- Your choice of additional spices

Cut the potatoes into thin, even slices. Drizzle a small teaspoon of olive oil on all the slices and then sprinkle them with salt and pepper and your choice of spices. (Try dill, lemon pepper or rosemary!) Microwave slices in a single layer on a microwave safe plate for about 2-3 minutes until they begin to brown (depending on potato thickness and microwave power). Turn over slices and microwave again for 2-3 minutes or until they start to crisp up around the edges. Remove, cool and enjoy your non-fried and guilt free potato chips.

Cheesy Spinach Delight (Serves 2)

Ingredients:

- 6-8 cloves of garlic

- 1 onion
- 10 small mushrooms (try baby portabellas)
- 1 bunch spinach
- Olive Oil
- Low-Calorie cheese

Chop the garlic into small pieces and slice the onions evenly. Cut the mushrooms and spinach into pieces, based on the size of your choice. Heat a tablespoon of oil olive in a sauté pan and sauté the sliced onions and chopped garlic until the garlic becomes fragrant (be careful not to burn!) Add the chopped mushrooms and spinach. Let simmer and cook for a few minutes, stirring occasionally. Add salt and pepper to taste. The mushrooms and spinach will cook down quite a bit. Once the mushrooms and spinach are cooked down, sprinkle some grated low fat cheese on top to give it that extra zing. Voila! You have a dish that's both high in taste and low in calories.

For a complete meal, increase the quantities of the ingredients and add a portion of whole-wheat garlic bread as an accompaniment.

Vegetarian Diet Tips and Tricks

- (This tip actually works well for anyone on a diet.) Maintaining a diet diary is an excellent way to keep track of your eating habits. You'll be surprised at the amount of food you eat and may even be shocked at the amount of unhealthy foods you ingest. Write down everything you eat (even gum!) for a few weeks and then go back and look over your notes. This will help you pick out what comfort foods you may be indulging and helps you to make a conscious choice to eliminate unhealthy foods moving forward.
- It is always better to sauté, roast, broil or steam food. Fried foods, even if they are vegetarian, lead to quick weight gain so use these cooking methods as healthier alternatives.

- Cheese is not always your friend. Yes, for vegetarians cheese is an easy snack but the fact is that cheese is typically 30% fat, which doesn't really help in weight loss. Make sure you keep your cheese consumption limited and in small proportions.
- Vegetarians tend to rely a lot on salads as meals, which is a very good habit because uncooked vegetables are a good source of energy and are extremely healthy. However mayonnaise, salad dressings and croutons used to give salads a more interesting taste tend to be high in fat so it is better to go easy on them or avoid them altogether. Mayonnaise can actually be up to 80% fat! Salads are very deceptive meals because we automatically feel that we're going the "healthy, weight-loss oriented way" and don't realize how high in fat and sugar dressings can be. Stick with olive oil and vinegar based dressings instead.

- Beans are excellent options for vegetarians on a diet. Lentils and beans tend to be high in fiber and protein rich and consuming them makes you feel full quite easily. Don't be afraid to experiment with canned beans as they help in making the cooking process much easier and convenient, but check those labels!
- Add artificial meat to your meal plan. When you go to a restaurant don't be surprised if you stumble upon an all-vegetarian menu that offers meat dishes. These are created using synthetic meats that replicate the flavor and consistency of real meat. They are excellent diet options for vegetarians, as they tend to be protein rich, low fat and generally have low cholesterol.
- As explained before, vegetarians may lack in certain nutrients that they would have generally acquired from different varieties of meat. Multi-vitamins can be essential in replenishing these nutrients.

- Snacks are an important part of a daily meal plan because all of us tend to feel hungry between meals and even more so when we're on a diet. The kind of snacks that you should indulge in should be "chewable" like low-fat cheese, baby carrots and tomatoes because they are healthier, low-fat options that satiate hunger and take longer to chew, causing you to slow down and enjoy what you're eating.
- Indulge in tofu. For ages, it has been an excellent substitute for meat and there are versions of tofu available on the market that has as few as 40 calories and 1.5 grams of fat. Tofu is very versatile and can be cooked in a number of ways to make it more delicious. Try stir-frying it along with exotic vegetables or cooking it up with different spices and wrapping it in wheat rolls. Use it to create healthy, low fat meals.
- Trying to lose weight doesn't mean depriving yourself of everything you love. Desserts are not

automatically the enemy and if you want to lose weight the sensible and reasonable way, ensure that you incorporate a treat or two into your diet occasionally. Choosing your dessert carefully is the best option, take a fruit like a banana or strawberry and dip it in low calorie chocolate or vanilla syrup and you're good to go. Another healthy option is low-calorie jam on a slice of brown bread or fat free flavored yogurt. This way you're literally having your cake and eating it too.

Veganism: Vegetarianism's distant cousin

Vegans are a class of people that follow the strictest form of vegetarianism. They do not consume any animal products or even by-products, like dairy products that are created using animal milk. Some strict vegans even avoid honey (because it is a by-product of bees). Vegan diets are difficult to follow but if done correctly it can help you acquire the skinny body you covet. (But remember – you still need to watch those calories!) If you are concerned with eating animal products and by-products, veganism may be right for you. Be sure to consult a doctor and get all the facts before starting a strict diet such as veganism.

Although vegetarianism and veganism can be strict diets, they are good options for trying to lose weight and they can also help you maintain your weight as well as help you to be healthier overall. Remember: these are not “cure alls” for losing weight – all factors should be considered first. These are just some options to help you in obtaining that skinny girl body you’ve always wanted, but keep in mind that you should choose what’s right for you and you alone. No one else can make these decisions for you – only you (and your doctor) know your body. Always keep in mind: it isn’t about torture. If something doesn’t feel right or you are having difficulty – it might not be the right path for you.

CHAPTER SIX: HOW BEING A SKINNY GIRL COULD SAVE YOUR LIFE

Looking great in your clothes is only one benefit of being a skinny girl. Type 2 diabetes, high blood pressure, heart disease, and stroke are more common in women who are obese. Obtaining your skinny girl self is about more than just looking great – it could save your life.

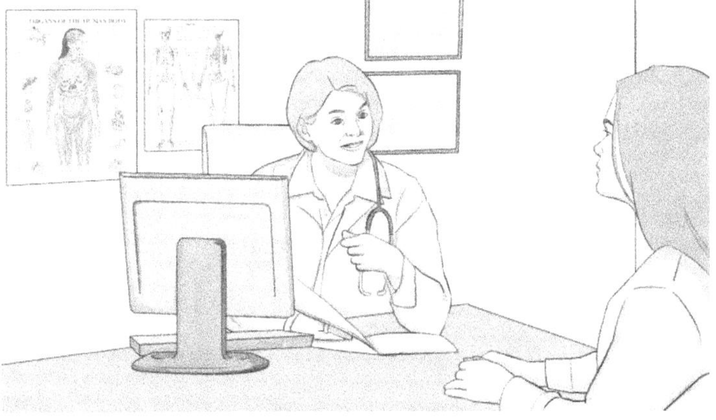

Being overweight brings with it a plethora of problems, the least of which is clothes that don't fit. People who are overweight or obese can develop health issues like sleep apnea, high blood pressure and even more life threatening diseases like Type 2 diabetes, gestational diabetes (and other pregnancy complications), heart disease, and strokes. Pursuing and maintaining a skinny girl lifestyle helps reduce these risks.

Type 2 and Gestational Diabetes: Protecting Yourself and Your Child

Type 2 diabetes is the most common form of diabetes. Many Americans have type 2 diabetes and may not even know it. Type 2 diabetes occurs when your body doesn't make enough insulin or your body doesn't know how to properly utilize the insulin being created. This condition is known as insulin resistance. Insulin is a hormone in the body that helps maintain the movement of sugars (or glucose) from the blood into the cells. Without insulin, glucose may build up in the blood and, in return, may cause your cells to starve from not having enough energy. This can cause health problems like damage to the nerves and small blood vessels of your eyes, kidneys and heart. It can also lead to a hardening of the arteries (called atherosclerosis).

Having too much glucose in the blood will cause a high blood glucose level, also known as hyperglycemia. This condition can eventually lead to kidney damage, heart disease and other health problems. Fat makes it hard for the body to use insulin, making it likely that overweight people will become insulin resistant.

Having diabetes is not fun. Symptoms of type 2 diabetes include feeling extremely thirsty, but with increased urination issues, as well as fatigue, dry mouth, nausea, numbness in feet and hands, skin infections and even blurred vision. In addition to not feeling well, it can be embarrassing when out in public to be constantly in need of a restroom. Outdoor hikes are almost impossible due to the lack of facilities and blurred vision may keep you from driving as well.

You may also have increased hunger, but lose weight. This might seem like a perk to some, but before cementing that idea, realize this: due to your body not using the glucose as it should means that your body will start using other fuels instead. As a result, you'll lose weight and extra fat, but you'll also lose muscle.

When people find out they have diabetes, it is normal to become disappointed and sad, but finding out you have this disease doesn't mean your life is over. Factors like the primary cause of your diabetes, how long you've had the disease, and how well your pancreas functions all determine how "curable" your diabetes is, but there are many good treatments to help at least lessen the symptoms.

Some of the primary treatments for type 2 diabetes are lifestyle changes, such as diet and exercise. Some doctors may recommend medications for more severe cases, but altering your lifestyle with diet and exercise is often the best way to treat type 2 diabetes symptoms and may even lead to a reversal of the disease. There are diabetic cookbooks and websites that can help you find recipes and offer suggestions on what types of foods are best to eat when managing diabetes.

Gestational diabetes is a form of diabetes that some women develop during pregnancy. Many women who contract gestational diabetes are often discouraged as well. Pregnancy is a time of hope and blessings for the future, but a sick pregnant woman is not the glowing ideal. Unfortunately, gestational diabetes really has no symptoms. Therefore, almost all pregnant women have a glucose-screening test between the 24 and 28 week period of their pregnancy (or earlier if you are at risk for diabetes). A woman with high blood sugar or glucose levels during pregnancy can be an indicator of gestational diabetes. More in-depth tests can be done for a more accurate diagnosis. When monitored closely, women with gestational diabetes have a good chance of having a healthy baby.

Here is one additional silver lining: woman who develop gestational diabetes during pregnancy do not continue to have diabetes once the baby is born. However, the chances of redeveloping gestational diabetes increase when or if you become pregnant again and this risk is increased if you remain overweight.

According to the *American Diabetes Association*, gestational diabetes occurs in about four percent of pregnant women and some studies suggest that overweight woman are almost two times as likely to get gestational diabetes. Women with gestational diabetes can pass the effects to the unborn baby and can cause the baby to develop hyperglycemia. Hyperglycemia can lead to macrosomia in the unborn baby, causing the child to become too large for the birth canal and may require additional assistance for delivery. This is often when a C-section is performed. If the child is born with hyperglycemia, it may have trouble breathing and may affect their heart function, which might lead to more time spent in the hospital after birth. Typically, these symptoms can be controlled and reversed for your child, but taking proper care of yourself first will help to avoid these issues from the start.

In summary, diabetes is not something to be taken lightly. Not only are you potentially harming yourself, but if you become pregnant, you could be harming your child as well. Fortunately, if you contract gestational diabetes, it will go away after nine months, but the effects on your child may be longer lasting. Changing your lifestyle and eating properly can help control and even prevent this disease. Don't you want that for yourself and your child?

How To Avoid High Blood Pressure, Heart Disease and Stroke

Ever wonder what those numbers mean when the nurse puts that annoying cuff on your arm? That restricting cuff measures your blood pressure – the systolic and diastolic. Ever get a bit worried when that same nurse says, "Let's take that again after a few minutes, okay?" That's because your numbers are probably a bit too high – 120 (systolic) over 80 (diastolic) is the norm and higher than that can indicate that you have high blood pressure, otherwise known as hypertension.

Your blood pressure is a balance of the amount of blood pushing against your artery walls. High blood pressure indicates there is too much blood pushing against those walls – just like too much water pressure in a hose. This increased pressure can cause risk of heart disease, including stroke and heart attack. Many people that have high blood pressure may not even know it, though common symptoms are severe headaches, fatigue, chest pain, a pounding in your chest, difficulty breathing and an irregular heartbeat. However, the best way to determine if you have high blood pressure is to have it checked regularly. Many people can have high blood pressure for years and not even know it until it's too late. Untreated high blood pressure can lead to other health problems, so it is best to get checked. Risk factors associated with high blood pressure are obesity, stress, drinking too much alcohol and a high salt intake. A lack of exercise may also be to blame. Once again, eating healthy, exercising, drinking less alcohol and maintaining a healthy weight (it's the skinny girl way!) can significantly reduce your chances of developing high blood pressure. These things can also help you manage your blood pressure once you've been diagnosed. Even if you think you are fine, too young, or not likely at risk, have your blood pressure checked at least once a year.

Heart disease consists of a variety of diseases that affect the structure or functions of the heart including narrow or blocked blood vessels, angina (chest pain), atherosclerosis, arrhythmia, stroke and coronary artery disease. The cause of atherosclerosis is a buildup of fatty plaque in your arteries that will eventually lead to the arteries becoming stiff. This can make it hard for blood to reach your organs and tissues. Atherosclerosis is a very common heart disease that can be caused by your lifestyle, obesity, diet and smoking. Damage from infections, heart attacks and even rheumatic fever can cause artery damage and lead to heart disease. Cardiovascular (heart) disease is the number one killer of all adults (both female and male) in the United States but can usually be prevented through a healthier lifestyle.

There are different symptoms of heart disease as well, depending on the type of heart disease you have. Some symptoms can include chest pain, numbness, weakness and coldness in your limbs. An unhealthy and fatty diet can lead to heart disease, but genetics may also play a part. Some people may be born with heart disease. Once again, as with your blood pressure, it's important to be in tune with your body and be an active participant in your care if you feel you may be at risk. Often, heart disease is not diagnosed until it is too late, after a person has had a heart attack or stroke.

According to the *American Stroke Association*, stroke is the third leading cause of death and the number one cause of adult disability in the United States. These numbers alone indicate that a stroke is very serious, but the reason for these statistics is due to the lack of proper treatment or prompt response when a stroke occurs. A stroke happens when blood to the brain is interrupted in some way. During a stroke, a part of the brain dies, due to lack of nutrients and oxygen. Early indication and action is crucial so that the stroke victim may recover some of their faculties and may even avoid death. Look for symptoms like sudden weakness or numbness in the face or limbs, sudden loss of vision, sudden loss of balance or a brief loss of consciousness.

There are different types of strokes and they are determined by what causes them. The ischemic stroke is caused by a clot in a blood vessel that keeps the blood from flowing to the brain. A TIA (a type of ischemic stroke– also called a "mini stroke") is caused by a temporary blood clot that restricts blood. A TIA can indicate that another stroke may be imminent and it is important to consult your doctor for further tests and evaluations. A ruptured blood vessel that causes brain bleeding is called a hemorrhagic stroke.

A stroke affects the brain, ultimately resulting in some changes in the overall body, such as slurred speech, vision problems, memory loss and paralysis. TIAs do not typically cause permanent brain damage, but ischemic and hemorrhagic do. Each type share the same symptoms, but differ in the duration (TIAs usually last for less than five minutes).

Immediate action (like getting to a hospital) after a stroke is the best way to recover, but additional treatments are available that can reduce the effects and permanent disability from a stroke. Medicines and medical procedures (like removing blood clots with the use of a catheter) are available as well to treat and prevent stroke. Some medications work by preventing blood vessel or clot formation. These medications can also remove clots from blood vessels. Managing your diet and avoiding other risks like a sedentary lifestyle and cigarette smoking, can reduce your risk of stroke. Exercising regularly, eating nutritionally good foods and getting regular checkups are the best forms of prevention.

Sleep apnea

Sleep apnea is a serious condition that causes you to stop breathing for a few brief moments during sleep. Pauses in your breathing caused by sleep apnea can last from a few seconds to a few minutes and can happen several times in an hour. Sleep apnea causes poor sleep quality and can cause you to be tired throughout the day. If you've ever slept next to someone when sleep apnea occurs you may have stopped breathing yourself!

Sleep apnea usually goes undiagnosed, and many do not realize they have it, because it occurs only in their sleep. The best way to diagnose sleep apnea is by sleeping with someone else present, so they can monitor you while you sleep. Be forewarned: you may also discover you snore loudly or talk in your sleep too! There are two different kinds of sleep apnea: obstructive and central. Although there are two types, you may experience a combination of both. The most common form of sleep apnea is obstructive. Obstructive sleep apnea occurs when the muscles in the back of the throat relax, causing your airway to narrow or close – causing an obstruction. This can cause you to periodically stop breathing. When the brain senses you are not breathing, it temporarily wakens you, so you can open your airways. This awakening caused by the brain can often go unnoticed. Central sleep apnea is caused by the brain not signaling the appropriate muscles to breathe. Central sleep apnea is less common than obstructive sleep apnea but has some of the same symptoms.

People who suffer from central sleep apnea are more likely to remember waking up briefly in the middle of the night than people who suffer from obstructive sleep apnea. Your risk of developing sleep apnea is increased if you are overweight, drink alcohol, smoke, or have high blood pressure (are you noticing a pattern?) Females are also less likely to develop sleep apnea, when compared to their male counterparts. Chances of developing sleep apnea also increase with age. Some symptoms of sleep apnea are loud snoring, pauses in your breathing during sleep and dry throat. One of the more common problems caused by sleep apnea is sleep deprivation and daytime sleepiness. Sleep apnea can go undetected in some, since symptoms occur mainly while you're asleep. If you think you have sleep apnea, consult your doctor as untreated sleep apnea can lead to heart disease and stroke.

Methods of diagnosis for sleep apnea in patients can include monitoring the person's sleep patterns, brain activities and other elements. Treatment includes lifestyle changes, surgery and breathing devices to use while you sleep.

Pregnancy complications

Obesity can cause pregnancy complications or gestational diabetes, as we've already discussed. Some of the additional pregnancy complications an obese woman can have include hypertension and blood clots. There is also a higher risk of having a caesarian birth (which could cause the mother significant blood loss) and of the baby being born with birth defects. Obesity can also lead to a higher risk of miscarriages or a baby being stillborn.

Preeclampsia is another condition that is common among overweight women. Preeclampsia develops during the late second or third trimester and is marked by high blood pressure and protein in a woman's urine.

To lessen the risk of a complicated pregnancy, women should try to maintain a healthy body weight prior to conception and gain only the recommended amount of weight during their pregnancy. Eating a balanced diet, moderating sweets and appropriate exercising while pregnant can help you avoid pregnancy complications and reduce your risks. Maintaining a healthy weight and living an active lifestyle can prevent your risk for diabetes, strokes, heart attacks, and even pregnancy complications. Remember to get regular checkups if you feel you are at risk for any of these life-threatening illnesses.

It seems like we've seen a pattern repeated quite a bit in this chapter – following a good diet with an active lifestyle can help you not only fit into those skinny leg jeans, but can also help you avoid some pretty serious health issues as well. Just another reason to start on the skinny girl way of life!

CHAPTER SEVEN: SKINNY GIRLS AND EATING DISORDERS DON'T MIX

Anorexia nervosa, bulimia and other eating issues can come into play when someone is focusing too much on their weight. It's not always about being too skinny though. This chapter discusses how to see the warning signs of an eating disorder, how to seek help and what to do if you know someone with these issues.

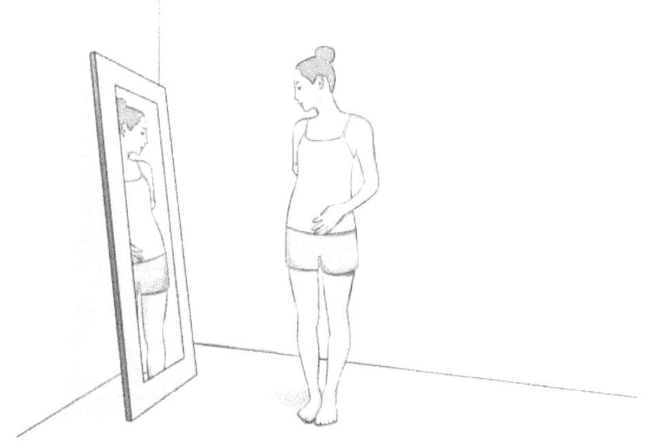

Although this book is discussing how to live a skinny girl lifestyle, we do not want our readers to resort to unhealthy ways to achieve that goal. There are well known, and serious, diseases out there that are caused by the desire to be thin. A variety of sources including the media, peer pressure and just an overall desire to be healthy sometimes contribute to these disorders. In this chapter, we'll discuss the most common sizes of women and how to determine if you or a friend has taken your weight to another level.

There are different sizes of women out there and some women may not even be aware of which category they fit. We've broken the most common sizes of women down into three main categories. There are skinny girls, medium (or average) girls and larger than life girls. With these three main groups, we can continue to break it down a little further.

Check out our chart below:

TYPES OF WOMEN	SUB CATEGORIES	DESCRIPTION
Skinny Girls	A. The Real Skinny B. The Average Skinny C. The Big	These women are what most people would refer to as skinny.

	Skinny	
Intermediates	A. Thin Intermediate B. Average Intermediate C. Large Intermediate	These women would be what most consider the "Average Woman." They are not skinny and not overweight.
Larger Than Life Girls	A. Grand B. Grander C. Grandest	These women are on the overweight to obese scale.

Some women are on the outer edges of these categories and may be larger or smaller than these sizes. If the women are smaller or larger than the sizes that are mentioned here, they may have an eating disorder or illness. In fact, it is difficult to diagnose an eating disorder just from the weight and physical appearance of any woman.

Many times these diseases coexist with other illnesses like depression, substance abuse or anxiety disorders. These diseases usually affect females more than males, and most commonly begin during the teenage years. Some people may start out with a desire to eat smaller portions to regulate their weight, but this regulation slowly becomes an obsession. These disorders affect people in different ways and can be broken down into several categories.

Anorexia Nervosa

Anorexia nervosa is one of the many eating disorders prevalent today and is common among teenagers. People with this disease are extremely afraid of gaining weight and have a distorted perception of their body weight/shape. Anorexics equate being thin with their self-worth. They may vomit after meals or misuse laxatives and diet aids in order to maintain an unhealthy and obsessive level of thinness. Most people with this problem may not be aware that they have a problem or may be in denial. Although they may already be very thin, their brain still believes that they need to lose more weight.

Anorexia nervosa most commonly begins in the teenage years and needs to be treated in the early stages of the disease. If it is not treated early on, lifelong problems can exist, or it can become almost impossible to overcome. If treatment is withheld for any reason, the person can suffer very serious health risks such as severe organ damage, brittle bones, osteoporosis and, eventually, even death. Very often anorexics are not aware of their extreme weight regime until someone encourages them to seek treatment. Since anorexia nervosa usually begins in the teenage years, it could be said that a large number of cases of anorexia nervosa are caused by social influences; those years are very critical for adolescents. Girls at that age are in an environment where people judge them solely on how they look and even make fun of them for it. In addition, our society and media often focuses on thinner model types as the epitome of a "beautiful" woman. This type of pressure can influence someone to participate in dangerous activities, such as anorexic eating patterns. Also, you rarely hear of anorexia nervosa beginning in elementary years. Younger children do not pay much attention to body image and may not even be aware of the ways in which they can dangerously alter their body. But once the pressures of team sports and school cliques enter the scene, this dangerous obsession can begin to take root.

Signs of anorexia can come in physical and emotional/behavioral symptoms. Physical symptoms include being abnormally thin, having extreme fatigue, insomnia, low blood pressure, and dry or yellowish skin. Emotional symptoms might be expressed as severe depression, irritability, a refusal to eat, societal withdraw and thoughts of suicide. In addition, a family history of this disease can contribute to the disease.

Oftentimes, people may mistake very, very skinny girls for being anorexic, but other symptoms must come into play in order to diagnose this illness. Some of the ways that anorexia nervosa is diagnosed is by checking to make sure a person's body weight is normal, taking blood tests and providing a psychological exam. Other tests may include x-rays, heart tests and checking of the organs function.

Anorexia can start as just a desire to lose weight, but can spiral out of control into a life-long, debilitating illness. Anyone who suffers from anorexia nervosa needs to seek treatment right away. If the person is severely underweight because of being anorexic, then it is most likely that they will require hospitalization. Treating anorexia nervosa can be long-term, depending on how long the person has been suffering with the illness. Anorexia nervosa has one of the highest death rates among psychological diseases. People who suffer from anorexia develop many complications, and their bodies are in terrible condition. Self-diagnosis or treatment does not work—consult the help of a physician.

If you do not feel comfortable talking to a doctor about your issue, or simply don't want to, seek out a loved one or someone you know who will help you seek advice and treatment and can encourage you throughout the process.

There is no specific medication for anorexia nervosa. People who are twenty-five percent below a healthy weight will need to be hospitalized in an inpatient program. The more underweight you are extends the time it will take for you to recover.

Treatment for people with anorexia nervosa includes plans to get the person back to a more reasonable and healthy weight as well as getting them psychological help. People involved in the treatment and recovery process may be psychologists, dieticians, a family doctor, family and friends. You can help a loved one by building up their self-esteem, encouraging them to seek help and providing ongoing support for their issue.

Bulimia

Bulimia is another eating disorder that people may confuse with anorexia nervosa as it contains many of the same habits and symptoms. With bulimia, people eat excessive amounts of food, often in a short amount of time, and then purge it later by vomiting, fasting or excessive dieting or use of diuretics and diet supplements. The main difference between anorexia and bulimia is that a bulimic person maintains a "normal" weight throughout the disease. It is often harder to diagnose a bulimic for this reason as there is often no physical aspect to alert others to the issue.

People with bulimia may eat excessive amounts of food to deal with stress or for comfort. After eating a lot of food they begin to feel out of control and this leads them to purge. After they purge –ridding themselves of all that food—they then start to feel guilty and the whole process begins again. It can be hard to detect bulimia in a person, because many who suffer from it have a healthy body weight. Most bulimics will binge and purge in secrecy, keeping this eating habit hidden from others. Some things to look for in a person you suspect is suffering from bulimia are someone who is eating excessive amounts of food without seeming to gain weight, going to the bathroom directly after meals, and exercising excessively. Another thing to notice is that bulimics may be secretive about their dining habits, preferring to eat food alone or even hide food. They may frequently talk about dieting or their perceived body image. Other people may begin to notice little symptoms in a bulimic person like dental issues, frequent trips to the bathroom and severe depression. This type of disorder can also lead to dangerous and serious health problems like dehydration, kidney failure, heart disease and, in some cases, even death.

Some of the main reasons for bulimia are the same for people with anorexia nervosa. If someone in your family has the disorder, it increases your chances. Having stressful jobs, that place importance on body image, such as athletes, ballerinas or gymnasts, can also increase your chances of developing bulimia. Social influences are once again another large factor.

Like anorexia nervosa, bulimia is more common during the teenage years and can last into adulthood. Bulimia is more common in females than males, another similarity it shares with anorexia nervosa.

People with bulimia can be treated with counseling. If you know someone who is bulimic, it is best to encourage them to seek help and let them know how much you care about them.

Bulimia is a long-term disorder and sometimes treatment can be unsuccessful. As a result, the individual can go back to being bulimic right after being treated. It's not rare for a person with bulimia to have to repeat treatment or participate in more extensive treatments again and again. Psychological therapy, medications and nutrition counselors are the most commonly used treatments for bulimia and will most likely need to be ongoing for the rest of the bulimic's life.

Binge Eating Disorder

Another eating illness is binge eating disorder, and it is the complete opposite of anorexia nervosa and bulimia. A binge-eating person eats excessively, not just once or twice (like many of us do on the holidays), but on a regular basis, causing them to gain excessive amounts of weight. Many people with this problem may only eat excessively when they feel stressed out and use food as a source of comfort, something to soothe away their sadness. People who suffer from a binge eating disorder may also be addicted to food and treatment is a good diet, exercise and a low stress life.

The difference from anorexia and bulimia is that binge eaters do not purge out the excess food they have eaten. The binge eater is not thin, but is overweight and usually obese. Although the exact causes of binge eating are not known, binge eating in many people is caused by their emotions. Many people with this disorder have sad or bad feelings, so they often turn to food for comfort. They may have been taught this coping mechanism, instead of other healthier ways, from their family. In their mind, the amount of food they eat will solve their problems, making them feel better about themselves. Food replaces those negative feelings with feelings of happiness. But only for a short period. In the long-term, it doesn't make them feel good, and can actually compound the negative emotions as weight continues to pile on. Then they turn back to binge eating to regain the good feelings and the cycle continues. Many have compared it to being addicted to a drug.

Some of us participate in binge eating from time to time. Have you ever had a really bad day where nothing was going your way, and you come home and eat all the junk food that you could? That is what binge eating disorder is like, except these people tend to overdo it a lot and, perhaps, every day.

As with anorexia and bulimia, it is important to seek medical and psychological help for this disorder. Prolonged counseling and learning about ways to cope better with stress can help the binge eater to kick this unhealthy and life-threatening habit.

More than just a weight thing

We have discussed the most common eating disorders above and gone into detail about their causes and symptoms. Now let's discuss the long-term effects that these dangerous eating disorders can cause on your body besides the weight aspect. These disorders might make you lose weight but these dangerous diseases can wreak havoc on your body if you allow yourself to get drawn into their web.

The Enduring Consequences

There is a possibility that individuals who suffer from anorexia are more likely to suffer from dehydration, painful kidney stones and, in extreme cases, even kidney failure and liver failure, which can lead to death. It may not even seem fathomable to someone that watching what they eat and being anorexic can lead to death, but it is the sad truth when the diet and purging is taken too far. Being thin in a healthy manner is definitely not a bad thing, but going about it the wrong way can lead to disastrous consequences.

With women, large amounts of weight loss can lead to menstrual problems to the extent that you may even stop getting your period and can lead to a condition called Amenorrhea, which may cause infertility and prevent childbearing.

Osteoporosis is a problem that is very deeply associated with eating disorders as lack of calcium creates a decline in bone calcium, causing bones to become brittle.

With bulimia, excessive use of laxatives and diet supplements to keep weight low, leads to a flushing out of potassium and sodium chloride from the body and can lead to electrolyte imbalance, which could lead to Arrhythmia. This irregular heartbeat syndrome could cause more cardiovascular problems and ultimately, death. Excessive use of laxatives could lead to dependence, meaning your bowel movements may never become normal and will only function if you use these laxatives.

Binge eating can cause a body to be more susceptible to different kinds of cancer, like bowel, breast and reproductive cancers as well as a heightened chance of getting diabetes due to the excessive intake of fatty and high-calorie foods on an ongoing basis. In addition, its effects on your mental state can be long-term, causing you to seek treatment for the remainder of your life.

Another dangerous result of binge eating is that you may have high cholesterol and high blood pressure problems along with increased triglyceride levels that may lead to the hardening of arteries causing heart diseases.

Is being overweight the new "norm?"

More common today is the growing trend of women who are overweight and don't think they are or don't realize it. There are a number of groups that fight for the right to be a "Plus Size" woman. While this is not necessarily a bad thing, some woman take this "right" to an extreme level—adding on weight and not knowing how much is too much. In a way, this is like anorexia in reverse. Anorexic girls don't think they are too skinny, and some overweight girls don't see that they are overweight. Sometimes this can start with a binge eating disorder.

While this problem with overweight women is not as common a problem as the issue for anorexic women, it can have just as severe consequences. In fact, this condition may be going unnoticed by the media and society because so many groups have spent years fighting back against the "be skinny" campaigns. In addition, the United States is a country of increasingly overweight people—so much that it is becoming the norm. In any country, the size of the occupants can be all over the map, but it's important to know the facts about proper weight loss and nutrition. If you or someone you know is struggling with weight and/or has feelings of depression, has a bad self-image or practices extreme dieting—please seek help. These disorders can be life-threatening and it is not worth risking your life.

If you need help please contact the

National Eating Disorders Association

Helpline at 800-931-2237.

CHAPTER EIGHT: ARE YOU ABOVE THE INFLUENCE?

Social media, television shows, advertisements and even fashion trends can influence even the most steadfast person. This chapter shows how even the most innocent of advertisements, perceptions, fashion and TV can sabotage a person. Learn the skinny girl secret to protecting your waistline and self-esteem from societal and media influences.

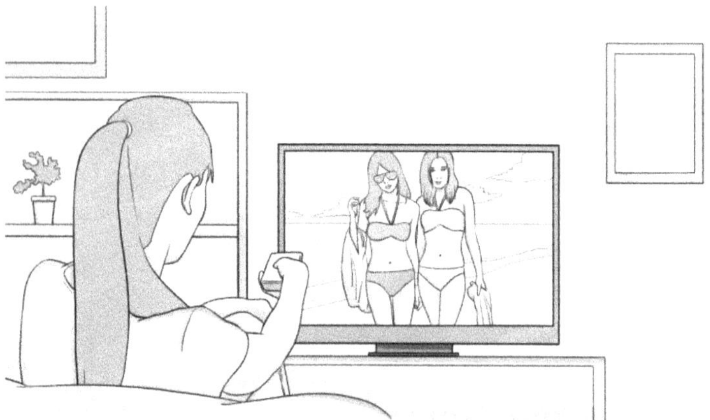

Societal and media-based influences tend to play off of each other in a very unhealthy way. What people see on television, read in magazines, and hear on the radio tends to influence their lifestyles. For example, a woman sees how her favorite celebrity dresses, does her hair and makeup and reads about the celeb's life on a weekly (or even more frequent) basis. She also sees the elaborate lifestyle the celeb lives and thinks, "I wish that were me!" Soon this woman changes her hairstyle and then maybe buys a few new pieces of clothing. The woman will begin to emulate the celebrity in appearance and will make changes to her own life, adopting a specific way of speaking, walking and even altering her entire lifestyle so it matches the celebrity she admires. Sounds pretty extreme, doesn't it? However, it does happen, but the degrees of intensity varies from person to person. Young people imitate the characters they see on their favorite programs. Young adults try to emulate their favorite reality TV stars. Just think back to when the TV show "Friends" first aired. Jennifer Aniston's character had a specific hairstyle that was emulated around the country and even given its own name, "The Rachel." It became one of the most popular hairstyles in history—simply because some famous actress wore it.

How people imitate what they see doesn't extend to just how they dress, their attitude or their beliefs. It can also extend to what they eat and their physical health.

Society's Influence On Our Weight

Society plays a large role in why some women believe that they are not overweight when they are. Most of the American population is overweight, so it may seem like the norm to some women. In fact, we have new terms from the media to describe being overweight: big, chunky, plump and "plus size" all make being overweight sound less significant than it truly is. If you come from a family of heavy people, have friends who are all large, or are overweight yourself, it may not seem like anything out of the ordinary.

But this is not a healthy trend, just like it is not healthy for anorexic girls to believe they are too fat when they aren't. Although accepting and loving yourself for who you are is important, being blind to your health can be deadly. It is not always just about the size. As we've stated in past chapters, you're overall health is the true key.

Some women may be overweight or obese and not acknowledge the health risks. Although any size woman can be beautiful, overweight women may ignore the risks their size poses to their health as a whole. As mentioned before, these women may never seek help for their problem, because they might not know or believe they have a problem. In the seventies, it was chic to be super thin, but now it's becoming more and more popular and acceptable to be overweight. But both types are extremes and the health risks are often not talked about—just the weight issue and how they look in a pair of jeans. This ignorance, in turn, can seriously damage a person's health in the long-term.

There is nothing wrong with loving your size and being proud of being a full-figured woman. In fact, loving yourself is a great thing, and I recommend it to everyone. But not being solely obsessed with your weight can be taken too far if you are putting your health in jeopardy. You don't have to necessarily lose all of your curves or all of the weight. Discuss your situation with your doctor and find out what an acceptable, healthier size for you would be and work to get there. Discuss all the health factors and risks. As we've stated earlier, being obese can lead to heart disease, diabetes and other life threatening illnesses. It's truly about the health of your body. Once you've reached your goal weight and have eliminated the unhealthy factors in your life, work to stay there. You can still be a beautiful, curvier woman without compromising your health. Don't give in to the societal influences around you—seek out your own answers.

If It's On TV It Must Be True

Let's face it. The media greatly influences the way women view their bodies. The world and media praise skinny women. We're bombarded on a daily basis with the "perfect beach bodies" and a plethora of perfect looking models on the cover of every magazine (mostly computer altered to look that perfect). Where does it all come from? The reason why being skinny is praised over being heavy is because it is healthier and traditional.

Women from earlier times were not as big as we are today. One factor may be the added chemicals that our foods contain and the easier ways we obtain that food. (Remember chapter 4?) Thanks to modern technology and knowledge, we no longer have to fight for our survival and can grow food in abundance. This is both a blessing and a curse, because with the increase of food stores, especially in the United States, comes an increase of waistlines.

However, there is also an increase in media stories and constant encouragement for women to lose weight. This is especially true because America has one of the largest populations of obese people.

As we all know, thin shouldn't "be in" if it is unhealthy. Being thin doesn't automatically mean you're healthy, just as being overweight doesn't automatically mean you are unhealthy. But all women should ignore the negative things that people put out there about their sizes and focus on bettering themselves. Only you (and your doctor) can determine what is healthy for you. Being overweight is not as bad as being obese, but for those women who still want to lose weight and get to a healthier, skinnier size then they should do so without feeling bad about it.

When it comes to the media, millions of women see commercials and magazines that influence them in their self-perspective. We have all seen the commercials that focus on dieting or losing weight. Products that promise to help us shed pounds, gadgets that guarantee a thinner you and workouts designed to be easy, but extremely effective. The only thing is that the men and women in these commercials are already skinny or medium sized. It creates an unrealistic standard. If you are overweight, it will take longer to achieve the thin standard that these men and women already possess. Even so, they are trying to lose weight. So why is this the case?

There has been some debate on this subject in many households, or people are at least thinking about this matter in their heads. Some people disagree with commercials showing skinny women trying to lose weight. They believe that it sends a negative message, a false claim, that can affect young women's images of themselves. If young women see skinny or medium-sized women on TV trying to lose weight, especially if the women are skinny or medium-sized themselves, they may start to get the impression that they are overweight—even if they are not. It seems like these women on TV are always trying to lose more and more weight when they already look thin. So how thin is thin enough?

On the other hand, some people agree with these commercials and say that showing a smaller-sized woman trying to lose weight shows that her diet has already worked to that point; she just needs to lose a "little more weight." However, once again, what constitutes as "thin enough?" When does it all end?

This can create an unhealthy cycle of dieting and exercise. This can be a downfall. There is no true calculation of how much weight was lost, where the person started from or when they stopped using the product. It leaves the consumer—you and me—unsure of what is the acceptable "thin" standard.

People also mention that showing an overweight woman on these commercials actively working on losing weight can be very effective, or more effective. But this is only true if they show many commercials of the same women. As the time goes by, people can see this same lady losing weight, and they can see that the diet is literally working. Today, with the advent of computer imaging and digital enhancements even this is hard for a consumer to determine. What is true? What is thin? As the consumer, you need to decide what you feel is best.

In addition, other commercials show thin, beautiful women doing glamorous activities and looking sexy while they are doing them. This can be depressing for overweight women and intimidating for skinny girls. The image on the TV can set a standard for beauty, and people accept it because they think, "If they're showing her on the TV and she looks that good, that must be what the ideal is." Or, "She has lost so much weight (assuming she had any weight to begin with) and she makes it look so easy! I want to be thin like her." Once again, the standard is based on what society shows us is the "norm"—not what our doctor or our health indicates it should be.

Traditionally the pressure has always been mostly on women. It is unfair for the media to ridicule women so much more than they do men. Overweight men need to lose weight just as much as overweight women do, but outside of doctors, most people just accept it when a man loses his muscular physique or gains weight.

Perhaps the most influenced people are teenage girls, who are also, hopefully, learning about proper health, body size and image in school. However, these two sources of information, one being based on facts and the other based on perceptions, conflict with each other creating confusion and misperceptions about health and weight loss. Naturally, most girls are going to look to their peers, the adults in their immediate life and society, to judge what is considered the norm. Again, as I have stressed repeatedly, loving yourself and your size is a great thing, but to be healthy while being lean is the best way to love yourself. If you have young girls in your household or sphere of influence—help them to choose the right foods and maintain a healthy weight. Be a healthy example to them and encourage them to reject the norms that society is pressing upon them.

Moving In The Right Direction

Although the media can portray unrealistic ideals, there are also many magazines and TV shows that present a positive image and influence. These magazines and shows praise women for trying to be healthy and living a healthier lifestyle.

There are also TV talk shows hosted by women who are not skinny, but of healthier weights (some are even overweight) that share their stories and struggles in order to help other women with their own body image issues.

In recent years, there have been numerous women encouraging overweight women to love their bodies and not despise them, especially famous women who do not fit the traditional ideal of perfect body weight and image. Their personal weight struggles have been aired in tabloid magazines, gossip columns, on the Internet and entertainment news shows for everyone to know about.

In my opinion, you should love your body and still try to lose weight if you need to. Appreciate everything you have and try not to take it for granted. You do not have to be bone thin to be healthy and you can still be unhealthy even if you're thin. In fact, most of the women that you see on television are not extremely skinny. Most of them are regular skinny or just naturally fit. (Sometimes television can make a person appear skinnier or larger than what they really are.) So basing yourself on them is an unrealistic and unfair standard. We cannot truly know how much a person struggles with their weight or health unless we walk in their shoes. It's important to make decisions about your health based on your own body and how it reacts.

Now I must ask: If it weren't for the media, would women have that same desire to be thin or be in shape? My personal conclusion is "yes," because they still learn from health professionals that being overweight lessens the quality of life and is a health hazard. However, social and media pressures contribute greatly to how we act on a daily basis and how we feel about our bodies.

So now ask yourself: Am I above the influence? Will I give in to the societal pressures of an unrealistic ideal—perhaps still being unhealthy in the process? Or can I chart my own course, with the help of my doctor, and maintain a healthy skinny body? It's up to you to decide—but I say Choose Yourself.

CHAPTER NINE: WHAT'S YOUR EXCUSE?

Do overweight women think differently than skinny girls? How can being an overeater start from childhood? Can fruit be bad for you? There are a plethora of misconceptions and excuses. Which ones do you hold tight to?

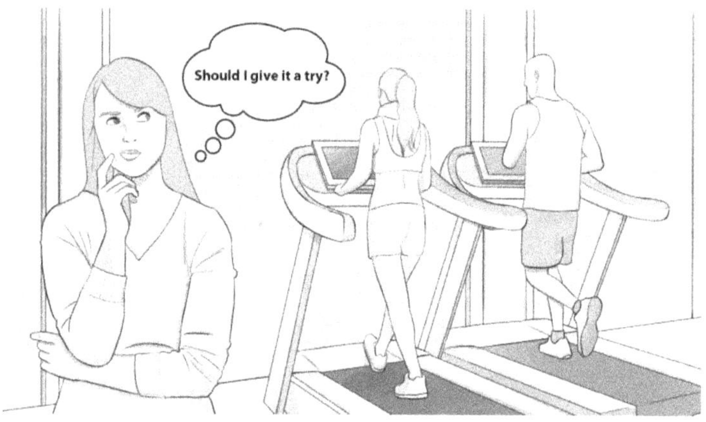

One of the most common mistakes some overweight women make is that they purposefully delude themselves. As we discussed in the previous chapter, some overweight women don't view themselves as overweight. Instead, they may use more "acceptable" terms like "medium size," "big boned," or "thick," (I've even heard "I'm just fluffy!") when in reality, they are simply overweight. No matter how these women view themselves, what silly terms they use or how they process the information, the important thing is that they eventually recognize that they are overweight and stop convincing themselves that they are not. Sometimes it will take a person outside of the situation to make this clear.

As we discussed in chapter 7, this situation reminds me of anorexic girls who are very skinny, but still don't think they are thin enough. Their problem is that even though they are where they should be weight-wise, they do not believe it and drop below the recommended, healthy level for their size. Their brains are not processing the information correctly, just like overweight women who think they are just medium size, do not process their information correctly.

We're not so different after all

Because our brains do not always process this weight information correctly (sometimes because of the social and media influences that we discussed in the last chapter occur), it sometimes takes an outside person to change our way of thinking. Someone outside the situation can tell us the truth. However, many people find it hard to be honest with overweight women, especially men. In fact, even if you ask a man to honestly comment on your weight, most will not. Most men are taught not to comment on a woman's weight. This politeness is ingrained in them from their mothers, sisters, girlfriends or wives. Although other people may find it hard to tell a woman she is overweight, her doctor will be honest, sometimes brutally, but for her own good.

Even though people may have a hard time telling a heavier woman she is large, there are overweight women who don't find it hard in the least to tell someone how skinny they are. They may even joke a little: "Do you eat?" or "You must not eat that much." They may even question you: "How much do you eat?"

or "Do you eat a lot?" or "You're so skinny…do you eat?"

Some skinny women may take this as a compliment; some will be offended by it, because indirectly, the person seem to be saying there must be a problem because you are so skinny. Many times, regular-sized or overweight women will tell a skinny girl how thin she is to her face and generally get away with it, but an overweight woman may get offended when the tables are turned. She may even have a word or two with you about it—possibly causing a fight. There is obviously a double standard here. Granted, some skinny girls can be very cruel, especially about overweight women. But if they are caught saying something outside their social circle, they suffer society's anger. It doesn't work the same when the situations are reversed.

At the end of the day, women will be women. We are sensitive and emotional creatures so even though something may be said as a compliment, it may not be taken as such. In addition, women can hold grudges and become spiteful if someone talks to them in a way they do not like. It is important to come from a place of love in all aspects with each other. If you believe a friend has a problem—either eating too little or eating too much—address it with them in the most loving and kind manner you can to ensure your message is heard properly. Also, be willing and open to hearing comments from your friends about your own weight issues—think about each comment carefully and examine where the comment is coming from before becoming upset.

Even though skinny women may sometimes become offended by the comments, they can often shrug it off. Many skinny women know deep down inside that many overweight women want to lose weight. Once again, it's important to treat each other with respect and have adult conversations. It is not for anyone else to comment on your weight—only for you and your doctor to decide. A skinny woman rarely comments on how overweight a larger woman is to her face, unless she is trying to be mean or is very oblivious. Many times a skinny girl will not comment because they have been in the overweight position and know what it's like. Some skinny women may even want to gain a few pounds, to be more of a medium size woman. But women rarely desire to be overweight. I have never met a skinny girl that wanted to become overweight. Think about that: how often have you seen a product on TV that promises to help you *gain* weight? It's always the other way around. The skinny girls that try to gain a few more pounds find it hard to gain weight. A fast metabolism or a high rate of physical activity, burning off more calories than what is consumed, may be the culprit against weight gain.

Before I move on, I know what you overweight girls are thinking: "Well, if a skinny girl wants to gain a little weight, all she has to do is eat. Just eat, eat, and eat." Well, not so fast, because she is thinking the same thing about you. She is thinking: "Well, if she wants to lose weight, all she has to do is stop eating. Just stop, stop, and stop." Makes you kind of mad, doesn't it? Because you know it's not that easy. For some of those skinny girls, it's not so easy to gain weight either. If it were, they would've been gaining their desired weight just like overweight girls would've lost their desired weight. It works both ways in many instances.

Excuses don't lead to success

Now, after all the talk about the benefits of women losing weight, let's talk about all the common mistakes and excuses women make.

Before continuing, I would like to mention that there are legitimate reasons that some women have a hard time losing weight, such as medical conditions. One such medical condition is called glandular disease, which affects the glands in the body and makes a person overweight. Having this disease can be very stressful, since a person is overweight due to a glandular problem and not a food problem.

Someone with glandular disease may also be upset and annoyed when people constantly accuse them of being fat from eating too much food and not enough exercise, when that is not the case. A glandular problem is a disease that is difficult to control and often cannot be helped by diet and exercise. You should be tested by your doctor to see if you have one of these disorders so you can properly adjust your lifestyle.

Many women (who do not have glandular diseases) claim it is too hard for them to lose weight and that's why they never really bother. Or they try for a week or two, get discouraged, and give up. How often have you heard a friend (or yourself) say, "I can't do it. My body aches from all the exercise and I haven't lost a pound!" It's true that it can be challenging to lose weight, but that doesn't mean you can't do it. Most certainly you can, you just have to increase your patience and not give up. It takes perseverance and persistence. It may not be easy to some, but it can be done.

Besides complaining about how hard it is to lose weight, another excuse women make is that they are not really fat, they just have "big bones." Sure, this may be the case for some women, although only about 15% of people are accurately listed as "big-boned." It is definitely not the reason you are fat, especially if you were not always big. Even if you are deemed as "big-boned," it typically will only account for a few pounds, not thirty or forty. In addition, even big-boned women can be a healthy weight. Heavy bones do not cause health problems—too much fat over the bones and muscles cause health problems.

Still another excuse that women make is that being big is in their genes. Their entire body is large, and they were born that way. Even if this is true, that doesn't mean you necessarily are going to be or have to remain large. It's just that you lived your family's lifestyle since you were born, or your family has allowed you to eat a lot of food without moderating its nutritional value. It could also be that you are used to eating a vast amount of food with your family for meals and snacks. You can change all that and get in shape. Take some time away from the family lifestyle and make your own, healthy, choices for one month. Did you lose weight? More than likely you did. Being born into a family of unhealthy eaters does not doom you to an existence of being overweight.

Using foods to celebrate events with your family is great. It is a natural thing to have potluck dinners, buffets, picnics and other festive events with your family, but you cannot blame them or that lifestyle for your continued weight problems. Once you became an adult, you were entitled to make decisions for yourself. It is now time to step up and make the decisions that will help you to be healthier. You can decide your own fate with a healthy balance of diet and exercise.

One common mistake women make when it comes to losing weight is to eat a large meal filled with unhealthy or fatty foods and then do some moderate exercise.

Tied into this mistake is usually the theory of: "If I have a diet soda, then this bag of chips is all right." They do not cancel each other out or balance the scale. You do not get to eat a bag of greasy chips, because you had a diet soda. The diet soda doesn't erase the calories from the chips.

This logic is flawed and can be traced back to the social and media inaccuracies we are fed on a daily basis. How often have you seen someone at the local fast food place order a large meal of greasy burger and fries, only to add a diet soda? Many people think that drinking diet soda is going to help them lose weight. It doesn't really work that way. (Although if you previously drank multiple regular sodas a day, you *could* see some weight loss initially.) To see real weight loss, you need to add in substantial exercise and other healthy eating habits. And by eating healthy I mean get the diet soda with a grilled chicken sandwich or a salad. Forego the large burger and greasy fries.

Changing what you think you know about weight loss

Some people who are trying to lose weight often skip their breakfast, feeling that they're making great strides in their diet by skipping an entire meal. The truth is, they're laying the groundwork for weight gain rather than weight loss. There are many good reasons why breakfast is said to be the most important meal of the day. One of them is that eating breakfast actually helps protect you from diseases. It also aids in strengthening your immunity so that you can fight the notorious common cold and flu. In addition, eating breakfast will help you not to overeat at your next meal—causing you to actually gain weight.

Most people eat dinner between 5 p.m. and 8 p.m., but breakfast is a whole twelve to fifteen hours away! That's a long time to not feed your body fuel and it slows down to conserve energy. The term "breakfast" is used because it literally breaks the fast that we are on post dinner and kick-starts our metabolism again.

Scientists also agree that regular breakfast eaters have more fiber and lower fat in their system and that a regular breakfast helps people to maintain their weight.

The Journal of American Diabetic Association published a study stating that women who ate breakfast daily were less likely to binge eat and have a reduced amount of calories than those who skipped the first meal.

An important thing to do while on a diet is to have a big, healthy breakfast so that you kick-start your metabolism after a long night of no food. Sometimes people drink fruit juices, eat fruit, cereals splashed in milk or have toast for breakfast. The truth is that these foods are high in fast carbohydrates and sugar, and are therefore not the best choice for having a healthy breakfast or for those wanting to get skinny. These foods break down quickly and do not have enough substance to get your metabolism going. Think about it: Have you ever had just a piece of toast for breakfast and felt hungry just an hour later? This is because the food breaks down too quickly in your body and doesn't provide enough fuel so you're hungry sooner.

Not all fruits are off limits though. Look for fruits with small sugar content and big nutritional value like raspberries, blackberries, apples and lemons. If you are a very adamant meat eater, the best options for you are turkey and ham. Again, stick with low sugar/salt and high protein options. Research shows the best breakfast foods are those that contain slow (or "good") carbohydrates and obviously, low, or no, sugar options.

For dieters, the best breakfasts include a combination of vegetables and eggs. Adding low fat yogurt, milk, tofu and cottage cheese is also favorable for those watching their weight. Strive to have a balance of protein and vegetables/fruits in each meal—starting your day off right with a good, balanced breakfast.

Another misconception women have when they are on a diet, is that they cannot eat any sweets. I find this to be untrue. You can still eat desserts while on a diet.

Of course, you have to limit your intake. By not eating sweets and denying yourself, you are going to fail. Remember what I said before about not torturing yourself? You will become miserable and you will soon go against your diet, causing you to start all over again. Even worse, you might even abandon your diet after feelings of failure. You may think, “This is simply too hard. I’ll never do it.” Nine times out of ten, you’ll indulge in sweets and possibly gain more weight than you initially started out with. Don’t restrict yourself too tightly and don’t be discouraged—be consistent and the weight loss and health will come.

There are plenty of delicious, healthy desserts you can try. One of the most natural sweets given to us on earth is fruits. Now, you’re probably thinking, “She just told me not to eat sweet fruits!” But they are okay in small quantities, but not to start off your day. Most fruits are naturally sweet. So the next time you have a sweet craving and want to satisfy your sweet tooth, try eating fruits like apples, bananas or some cherries. I know it can seem confusing, but do a quick internet search to see which fruits are best and strive to add those to your diet.

Another mistake people make starts out when they are young. Have you ever sat at the table with family and someone told you that you can't play or be excused unless you finish all of your food? This is a common, old-fashioned rule that can sometimes be taken to an unhealthy extreme. Some parents or guardians will give their children more food than what the child can actually eat and force the child to eat all of it. If children do not finish all of their food, they are often punished. Being forced to clean your plate when you were young began an unhealthy habit that probably continued well into your adult years. Do you have trouble stopping when you are full? Do you clean your plate even when the food isn't good? This can be a sign that eating is simply a habit for you and indicates that you do not have healthy eating habits. Work to break this cycle, especially if you're having trouble losing weight. One way to combat this is to use smaller plates and give yourself smaller portions that are more easily consumed.

In some cases, this “clean your plate” mentality can lead to childhood obesity. Most parents or guardians are not aware that they are planting the seeds of what could become a lifelong bad habit. They just think a child should eat all of their food. They may think the child is just being stubborn, when, in fact, they are just full. They are not aware that they are over-feeding their children. If you are a parent whose child is obese, consider this advice. There is a possibility that you are over-feeding your children. Talking with your doctor or doing simple research will help you determine how many calories your child should be consuming each day. Childhood obesity is becoming a huge problem, and you as a parent, have the power to stop your child’s obesity in its tracks. If you do not educate yourself and your child, you are only contributing to this issue. If this habit is continued, childhood obesity will grow with your child into adulthood. If that isn't reason enough to take preventative measures to teach your child about healthy eating habits, consider the fact that most obese children suffer from low self-esteem. These kids are often bullied and can carry these issues into adulthood. Preventing obesity, low self-esteem and adulthood health issues can start at your dinner table. Act now.

There are so many misconceptions, lies and bad habits in our world today, it's time we took back our lives and our health. Start educating yourself, loving yourself and one another and get on the road to the skinny girl life you've always dreamed about. The time to start is now.

CHAPTER TEN: BREAKING DOWN THE FAT

Even if you are healthy and thin, everyone should care about the growing obesity epidemic in the United States. Obesity is growing in number and affecting all of us. This chapter breaks down what it means to be obese and what is being done to combat this serious health issue.

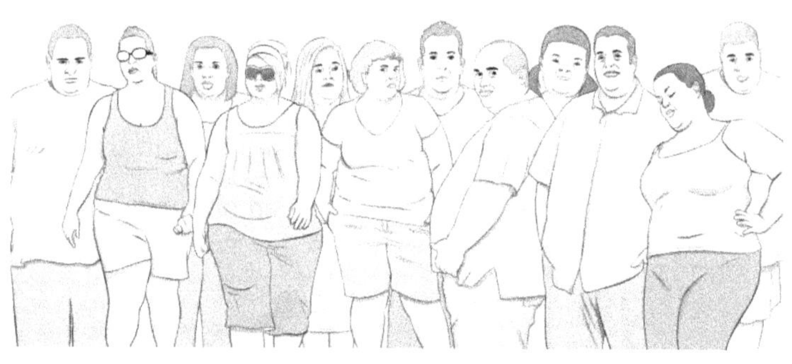

Americans seem to have food in abundance. It seems easy for Americans to obtain food. But, I bring this up because there seems to be a great amount of homeless or poor Americans living in poverty or near poverty. Surprisingly, some of these people are overweight. If the homeless can't afford to pay rent or the mortgage on homes, where is the income for food coming from? Where is the food coming from? Could it be that they were overweight before becoming homeless? One obvious, plausible answer to these questions is this: Government Assistance. Some people living in poverty or near poverty may be on some form of government assistance and often buy what is affordable, but affordable does not necessarily mean healthy. We discussed in earlier chapters how junk food is cheaper and more easily accessible than the healthier alternatives. It is cheaper to buy a can of green beans loaded with sodium and other preservatives than it is to buy the same amount of fresh green beans. It's easier to buy a sodium, calorie and grease-filled item off a dollar menu at one of the various fast food restaurants dotting our landscapes than to get a grass-fed or organic burger.

The same principle applies to people who are not on public assistance, but have limited amounts of money they can spend on food. It may be cheaper to live off a dollar menu at a fast food place than to buy a day's worth of groceries. Therefore, people at the poverty level could be unhealthy and even obese, even if they aren't eating a lot of food, because they are eating the wrong kinds of food.

You bought it. You eat it.

No matter what the case may be, it seems that Americans have food in abundance. For example, have you ever gone to a restaurant, ordered a dinner, and the plate contained more than what you could eat? You ordered a hot dog and some fries, but the serving size was enough for three people. Have you seen those food shows that get excited about the huge burger challenge or the burrito the size of your head? We're always looking for the best deal. Buffets and "All-You-Can-Eat" places are popular because we're getting more food for your ever-stretched dollar.

Some people will eat all of the food on these overstuffed plates, so they don't waste any money. Have you ever heard someone say, "I got bread, salad, a huge steak AND dessert for only $12!" They are happy to get more for their money. Who can blame them? They just want to claim everything they paid for, or they might feel bad about spending the money and not eating everything. Even though we didn't ask for that much food, we feel obligated to eat it all so our $12 doesn't go to waste. This "obligation" type thinking may be causing Americans to become overweight or even worse, obese.

Too many Americans feel like they are obligated to finish their plates, even if they don't want to and even if they are already full. Were you taught to finish your plate as a child? We talked about this in the last chapter—you could be eating all that food just out of *habit.* Women should only eat until they are satisfied.

This doesn't mean stuffing yourself, it means knowing when you're comfortably full. When you've eaten *just enough*. A good rule of thumb is to know that it is okay to leave a bit of food remaining on your plate and to train yourself that it is all right to walk away from a plate that isn't empty.

How fat is too fat?

I have spoken to some of my skinny friends on several different occasions about eating three meals a day. Many have mentioned that they don't eat three full meals a day. We each look at this as normal. If this was mentioned to some people, some of them will conclude that we have eating disorders, when we really do not. We eat when we are hungry and that is it. Sometimes we're still full when the next standard meal time comes around, so we skip one meal. It doesn't mean we have an eating disorder. Why eat more if you're still full? Being full, or not hungry, is your body's way of saying it does not need any more food. Learn to listen. It makes me wonder why some overweight people eat more than three full meals a day and what is wrong with that picture. Are we living in a society that praises overeating with little to no exercising?

Another thing I have found is that whenever I see a different doctor or nurse, they each have a different mindset about things. For example, if I were to go to a doctor that was skinny like me, they would tell me that I didn't need to gain any weight, that I am fine at my current weight level. On the other hand, if I were to go to a nurse who was overweight, she would tell me that I need to gain some weight. Other girls in my situation have told me similar stories with their doctors and nurses.

In my opinion, doctors and nurses may be misleading some people because of differences in personal opinion. So I pose this question: Who would you take advice from when it comes to concerns about eating healthy or losing weight? The doctor and nurse that are in good physical shape or the doctor and nurse that are in poor physical shape? You do the math. I'm not saying that you shouldn't seek the advice of medical professionals. It is very important to see healthcare professionals for your physical and mental well-being. Just pay very close attention to what they are telling you. If something doesn't sound right, then maybe it is time to seek the advice of another professional.

Remember that no one is perfect, and anyone can make mistakes and give you misleading information. If your health professional gives you advice you do not think is appropriate, seek a second opinion or ask for tests that will determine your overall health. As we've stated before, it's not all about your weight.

What's weighing you down

We have discussed obesity and being overweight in terms of the body mass index, but never actually covered what obese is in a way that is easy for everyone to understand.

A person falls into the obese category if they are more than 20% over their ideal weight (according to the BMI and taking height, age, sex and build into account.) Being obese also means to be so heavy or morbidly overweight that you may be putting your life at risk. The activity level of obese people is typically very limited, and some will utilize large wheelchairs or motorized scooters when they are out in public instead of walking. This is because they are unable to walk due to their mass. The extra weight puts stress on their muscles and joints, creating pain. Some obese people will not or cannot go outside of their homes and may not even be able get out of their beds due to their size. Some overweight people are able to hide the fact that they are overweight, because of their build or height. But it is hard not to miss a person who is obese.

Being overweight indicates that the person is over what their body mass index recommends, but it is not enough to put their life in jeopardy with their size. They can move around fairly normally, though they get winded quicker than a fit person. On the other hand, an obese person may have to slow down more often than slender people and, as stated, may use transportation devices to get around. Unfortunately, these devices only continue to contribute to the issue, enabling the already obese person with even less physical activity. Obese people may have disorders (as we discussed in chapter 7) that cause them not be able to control their weight, and others are simply eating themselves to death. It can be hard to tell the difference, unless that person tells you directly. Either way, by a disorder or by eating, they are at risk for an early death. Their bodies and organs, much like their joints and muscles, cannot handle the strain of supporting that much weight. Over time, their body will shut down from all the excess pressure.

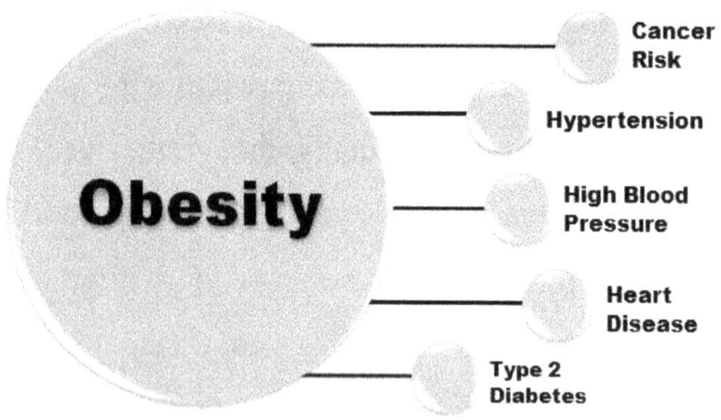

According to the CDC, currently around one third of adults in the United States are obese, and 12.5 million children between ages two and nineteen are obese. This rate will only climb if we, as a society, do not take note and make the necessary changes.

Reversing the trend

Throughout America, as the rate of obesity becomes more and more alarming, there are some people and organizations taking up the fight against obesity. They are fighting obesity in both adults and children. "The Healthy, Hunger-Free Kids Act of 2010," introduced the Child Nutrition Reauthorization Bill, which provides funding for federal school meal and nutrition programs. This allows the USDA to set standards for foods that are sold in schools and gives funding to schools that meet the new nutritional standards. This helps fund breakfast and lunch programs that are healthy and nutritional—not only helping kids eat better, but also assisting low-income children to have a meal that they might not otherwise get. The act also helps communities to establish farms and gardens for the schools that support the WIC program.

Adults are fighting obesity the same way children are. Communities all over the country are starting up programs geared toward educating adults on how they can combat the risk of obesity by providing information on healthy foods and explaining the benefits of physical activity and awareness.

While the programs can work, the problem lies in adults and children not implementing these initiatives outside of the programs. In addition, it's important for people to make these changes on their own and without the government overstepping their boundaries. Parents have to want to help themselves and their children to be healthy. Providing them with education about proper eating and nutrition is the first step toward those healthy goals and in curbing the obesity trend, but each individual person must continue to take up the fight.

Obesity is an unhealthy trend occurring in the United States, but with the right programs, education and sources for nutritional food, people can begin to buck this trend and get back on a path to healthier eating. It is never too late to start eating better—even if you can't move much now due to your weight. Take the first step, make better food choices and start your journey.

CHAPTER ELEVEN: SOCIAL EATING EFFECTS

Have you considered that your extra weight may not be genetic, but cultural? Are your friends and family making you fat? This chapter shows you how to carefully examine the long term effects of certain family/cultural perceptions toward food.

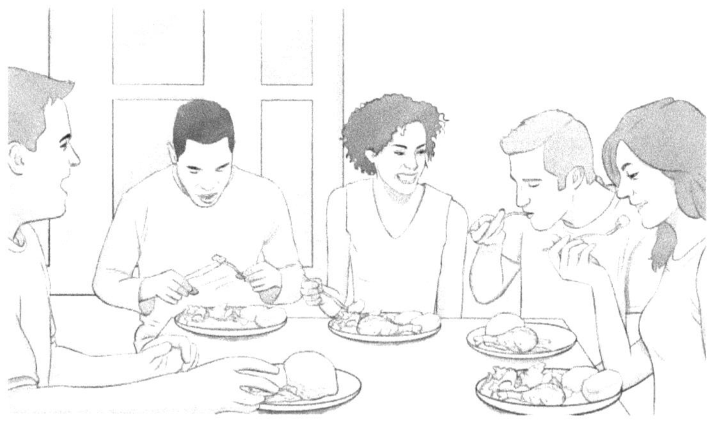

As mentioned earlier, society and the media can have some very bad effects when it comes to women and their weight issues. Television, social media and even social eating can have an effect on how we eat and what we weigh. Although the media taunts us with delicious new food and never-ending food buffets, they also sell us weight loss products. It can make for some pretty confusing and conflicting emotions. In addition, our friends and family can impact how we eat as well. We all love getting together with friends to socialize and have a great time. Often it's around the buffet, dinner table or other social eating event. Social eating is eating out with friends or family, or eating with them in their homes. Social eating also takes place when eating out in public—with or without friends.

Food is not a bad thing in itself. We have discussed how making healthy food choices can help us to maintain and even lose weight and food is a necessary source of fuel for our bodies. But when surrounded by other people, even though they are friends and family, we often make poor food choices and this effects whether or not we gain or lose weight. People can also have positive effects on our food choices—depending on who you surround yourself with, the bonds you have with them and their perspectives as well as your own. If you are usually steadfast and firm in your own opinions and actions, then you won't be too easily influenced. If you tend to fall in line with everyone else, you're going to have a harder time.

We often get together with friends or family to share special occasions like Christmas and Thanksgiving. Celebrations are fun with great big, elaborate meals and everyone pitching in to make the feast. It is a bonding time. Being together with family, cooking, and contributing to the meal is a lot of fun. But sometimes, if you are trying to eat healthy, you want to avoid the not so healthy foods, like gravy and heaps of mashed potatoes. You certainly don't want to sit at a table loaded with everything you've been trying to avoid, such as apple and pumpkin pies or homemade Christmas candies. At family events like these making healthy food choices can be hard (or downright impossible) because you don't want to offend someone or drive yourself insane between resisting temptation and overindulging.

Family and their influence

Our choices can offend some people, even family members, if they do not understand we are trying to watch what we eat and we want to lose some weight. They might just think you're being picky. Or they may think that you are being selfish by not putting off your diet for "just one day" to enjoy the meal. (How often have you heard that one?) No one wants to tell Aunt Edna that her triple fudge chocolate pie isn't healthy and it's especially hard to restrain yourself when Aunt Edna herself is pushing the piece in front of you.

If you don't want to offend them, you may eat more than you originally intended to and may eat the foods you were originally trying to avoid. After all, Aunt Edna brought two other pies…don't you want a piece of those as well? Now you've eaten three pieces in addition to your already overloaded plate! Not only do you feel stuffed, your healthy eating plan has fallen to the wayside.

At times like these, if you eat more than what you wanted or if you eat things you didn't want to eat, you may feel guilty or bad for cheating on your diet. If you chose not to eat you may also feel bad or guilty for hurting someone's feelings, and you may quit your diet altogether. It seems to be a no win situation and a vicious cycle. If you did reject someone's food you may have also been subjected to comments from your family such as, "Oh come on! It's just one day! You're already too skinny!"

What do you do if you have family or friends who make comments that you are too skinny and push you to eat more than what you are comfortable with? They are not trying to hurt you on purpose, but they might hurt you accidentally without even realizing it. So what can you do?

You need to be strong and stick to your eating plans as much as possible. Let them know in advance about your eating habits, and if you are on a diet. Be firm, but nice in how you approach the event. If you can't talk with everyone prior to the day, just say, "I'd love to try just one small piece of my favorite," and then pick one of Aunt Edna's pies—not all three—and have just one bite. (Chances are she'll be too busy trying to get others to eat her pie that she won't notice you only ate a small portion.) If you're not too skinny and are on a weight loss program, then let them know it. Make sure to thank them ahead of time for being understanding about you trying to maintain, lose, or reach your desired healthy weight. To lighten things up, you can playfully tease that you are trying to live a long, healthy life, so you can visit them more often (and eat small portions of their delicious food). Keep a lighthearted attitude and your family and friends will respect your decisions and may even ask you to help them in their weight loss journey!

There are two ends to the family spectrum when it comes to dieting. On one end, your family might think you are fine the way you are and try to stop you from dieting. On the other hand, your family might encourage you to lose weight. Family can be especially hard on a woman who is trying to diet, whether they mean to be, or not.

Mothers often seem to worry about you not eating enough and can make it difficult for a woman to lose weight. They may say that you're worrying over nothing and that you're perfect the way you are. While we all love our mothers, (and you are great no matter what you weigh) but sometimes they don't see us how we really are or may not understand the health issues plaguing us. I'm sure at one time or another, we have all been guilt tripped into something by Mom. After the fact, we find ourselves shaking our heads for listening to them.

Various things a mom will say to stop her daughter from dieting if she doesn't think it is necessary include: "You're beautiful just the way you are…" Then there's the other infamous line: "You're not fat," and one that's guaranteed to cause a flinch: "You get your build from me. Are you saying I'm fat?" The first two sayings are nice; it is how our moms say they love us, no matter what we look like. But the last one, and others like it, can cause us to stumble on our weight loss journey.

For a family that encourages you to lose weight, it can go two ways. They can be a positive, driving force that supports you in your quest to reach a healthy weight. Or they can be the reason you are on a diet in the first place. A family that supports your decision and helps to motivate you is a blessing. A family that tells you that you need to lose some weight can be a mixed blessing. A family that says you're fat and does it frequently can be a curse and may even be causing your weight issues. How we speak to one another can cause significant impact on our health and weight, sometimes causing us to eat more to sublimate other feelings.

If you come from a family where it seems like everyone but you is thin, that can be another negative motivator, even if they don't comment on it themselves. You may want to fit in better with your family and feel like an outsider. Maybe even your family comments if you take even the smallest bits of food because they think you can't control yourself. Or they try to pacify you by saying you aren't fat, when you know you are. They are only trying to help, but too often, can be hurting your progress.

Friendly Influence

Eating with friends can be like eating around family. They can say some of the same things that family say, especially if you've known the friend for a long time. Then again, it can be a whole new ball game. It ultimately depends on what kind of personality you have and how close to your friends you are.

Eating around friends who constantly comment on how many calories they can eat, or who opt only for waters and salads, can make it awkward and uncomfortable for you to eat with them. Ever have that friend who only orders water, but then stares at your chicken salad like she's starving to death? While you want to lose weight, trying to eat around people who constantly talk and worry about it can make the whole thing uncomfortable. Worse, they may even start to comment about your calorie intake and offer advice that is meant to be helpful, but instead winds up being overwhelming and discouraging. Remember, it's not about torturing yourself in any way and your journey is different from anyone else's. You need to do what's best for you. Use the knowledge you've learned in this book to help your friend make better choices too. Or, better yet, buy her a copy and get into a healthy routine together!

We can also pick up on our friends' habits and attitudes toward dieting. If a close friend has a casual attitude toward healthy eating and exercising, we might find ourselves adopting the same attitude. If the friend is gung-ho about exercise and eating healthy, and is on a strict diet, we might adopt that person's attitude and regimen. I have a friend who always wants to get appetizers to share when we eat out, but then I end up eating most of the food!

Adopting another person's food attitude can be both a good thing and a bad thing. Losing weight is fine, but do it responsibly and reasonably. Otherwise, it will backfire on you in the form of gaining back the weight, injuring yourself or inadvertently depriving yourself of something you needed. You may not even realize what's happening. What is important is that we make up our own minds and do not apologize for it. We have to set our own standards for healthy eating and exercising. It's best to say, "No thanks," ahead of time before being caught with the nacho chip in your mouth. It is good to get advice from our friends, as they can be a great form of support in terms of encouragement and motivation. However, we also have to do what works best for us.

If your friends are supportive and positive about your dieting regime, then you have great friends and should tell them so. If your friends are skeptical and make remarks that hurt your feelings or make you think dieting is a bad idea, then you might want to evaluate your friendship.

Public influence

When a woman is dieting, there is nothing like eating in a public place to make her feel self-conscious. When she orders her respectably healthy meal and a diet soda to go with it, she feels like everyone in the room knows why she's eating a grilled chicken breast with honey mustard sauce on the side.

Chances are this is your own perception and not the reality. There really aren't that many people paying attention to you. In fact, they are probably thinking the same thing you're thinking: "What does that person think of my meal?"

Perhaps you are overweight and fear that people will judge you for your food choices. If you are self-conscious about eating in public, you might go to extremes and simply order a plain salad with no dressing and a glass of water, then only pick at it. (Now you're the girl drooling over someone else's plate!)

In the end, you will only end up binging in the privacy of your home to satisfy your appetite. Order yourself something healthy, in moderate proportions. If that is not possible, then trim off what you cannot eat. Don't think you shouldn't eat, but instead, simply enjoy your meal and don't worry about what others may be thinking. Maybe they are thinking, "Wow, I wish I had her willpower!"

Finding the Support You Need

Dieting is difficult for some individuals. It gets even harder for people who cannot understand why they chose to diet or those that cannot comprehend why being a healthy size is so important. Everyone has different priorities and backgrounds and many factors effect dieters. Adding judgmental or critical people to the mix, may further complicate your weight loss journey.

If you are related to a dieter or are friends with one, you may get irritated with their obsession to lose weight and eat healthy but remember eating healthy is fine and people struggling with weight issues are super sensitive. Those embarking on diets for the first time might get moody and irritable and this is when they need support the most. Be aware of the struggle that your dieter friend is going through and make every effort to support them in making healthy life choices without being critical. If you are a dieter, it is important that you find solace in a group of like-minded individuals who understand why being a smaller size is so important to you. In fact, even better than just looking for friends and family to support you is to actually go out there and join a dieters support group to ease you into a diet oriented lifestyle, if you are trying to diet for the first time. People find solace in groups that understand their struggles.

No matter where you are on your weight loss journey, it's important to surround yourself with people who understand and encourage your goals. Be firm in your desires and communicate to the people in your life so they can also understand where you are coming from. Once again, this is your body and your dream to be a skinny girl. Only you can make the choices needed to obtain that goal.

CHAPTER TWELVE: ACCOMPLISHING YOUR GOALS - ONE STEP AT A TIME

It's time to discover what it is that motivates you. How can you find the motivation to keep going and not give up in your weight loss journey? This chapter will give tips and advice about how to stay motivated and where to find encouragement for your success.

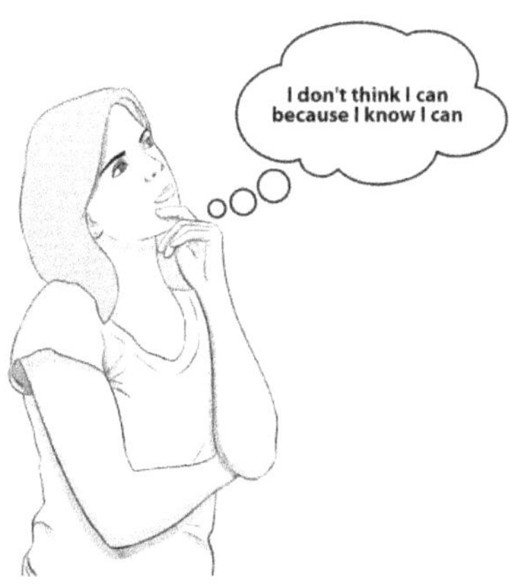

Millions of women in America are trying to accomplish similar goals. Marriage, kids, and careers make up the majority of the goals women strive to achieve within their lives. Another one of the main goals of women around the country is losing pounds to reach a healthy, standard weight. Unfortunately, many women do not accomplish that goal for a variety of reasons. Some reasons women fail to stick to their diets and lose weight is due to the lack of support and motivation. Many may simply become bored with their diets. Believe it or not, some women try to gain weight and find it hard to do so. In fact, it may be harder for some women to gain weight than it is for some women to lose weight.

No matter what the circumstances are, every woman who is trying to lose weight must never give up on their goal. Think about your health and your future, and think about the people around you, especially the ones that depend on you. Wouldn't it be great to have more energy for your husband and kids? Life is so much easier and enjoyable when you are living it healthily.

Perks to losing weight

If you are overweight, then you already know there are some things that you cannot do comfortably, or may not be able to do at all. You might walk up a set of stairs and find yourself having to stop about halfway through, just to let your heart rate get back to normal. You stop midway and you're sweating up a storm and generally feeling horrible. Then you head up the rest of the steps and wind up taking another break at the top, because you're out of breath again.

Then there are the times you play with your children. Do they exhaust your energy quicker than they exhaust their own? Wouldn't it be nice to keep up with them and be able to play with them for longer periods? Instead, you're sitting on the couch watching them have fun without you. Life doesn't have to be lived this way.

Maintaining a healthy weight will help you enjoy life to the fullest. You'll be able to breathe easier, more naturally and move faster. The sluggish nature will be gone. You'll be able to climb those stairs in one go without having to stop or feel winded. You will be able to do things physically that you could not before and accomplish more demanding tasks. Being physically fit will open up a whole new world of activities and experiences.

Your diet is your diet.

If you're going to lose weight and achieve your goals you must not give up. I cannot stress that enough. It is a lot easier to give up than to lose weight (as anyone who has tried dieting before can tell you), but you have to keep your goals in mind in order to keep going. Think about playing with your kids, enjoying more activities with friends or simply feeling better to keep yourself motivated.

Also, be patient about losing weight. Unless you are just trying to drop a few pounds or less, you're not going to lose all the weight you want in just a week. Losing weight is a process and takes time. Nobody loses all their desired weight in a month and then keeps it off. You didn't add all the weight on overnight—don't expect to take it off that quickly either! Be patient, follow your diet and keep moving forward.

For some people it can take as little as three to six months, or maybe even less, to reach their desired healthy size. For others, it can take a few years or more to lose weight, but remember you always have to be patient. Don't compare yourself and your progress to other people. Everyone loses weight differently. Focus on yourself and your goals only. The more you work on your diet, and the fewer times you give it up, the quicker you will lose weight.

Motivate yourself with fun

One great way to stay motivated is to have a friend or group to share in the process. Having someone who is dieting alongside you is a great way to receive and give encouragement and maintain motivation. Doing anything alone can at times be depressing for people. Dieting is hard enough as it is, so finding an exercise buddy or joining a group can take away some of those feelings of loneliness and make your diet easier to stick with. Also, try to find fun ways to lose weight, such as taking dance lessons or (if you're self-conscious about dancing in public) even just dancing to your favorite songs in the privacy of your home. If you are shy, or feel self-conscious about dancing in front of a large group, you can even arrange for private lessons. As your confidence increases, you may eventually participate in group classes. Not only is this a great form of exercise, but you will also learn a new, fun skill and you will acquire a hobby that may stick with you for the rest of your life.

Create fun, active games that allow you to move around a lot, or fall back on some enjoyable childhood games. Do you remember racing your friends to see who could get to the corner first? Or what about playing tag? Being an adult doesn't mean you can't engage your friends in these amusing and lively games. Whatever games you do decide on, make sure they are games that will get you up and moving. Have fun, but also remember you're trying to lose weight, so get that body moving!

Getting involved in sports can be another enjoyable, physically active way of losing weight. Some companies have softball teams their employees can participate in and anyone who has the opportunity to do this should consider it. Not only can it be a way of losing weight, but it can also help you meet people and build friendships. It can be a huge self-confidence booster too.

Another way to stay motivated and encouraged is to seek the help of a personal fitness trainer. A personal trainer can be very rewarding and sometimes very demanding—pushing you more than you would yourself). If you can get a professional, quality trainer to help you with a weight loss program, you are more apt to stick to a program and, consequently, lose weight.

Make sure that you look for a personal trainer that is knowledgeable and one that will help you on your journey to losing weight. You want someone who is going to be your partner in your goals, someone who will motivate, encourage and even demand you go that extra mile.

An alternative to the personal fitness trainer is to find a class or group at your local gym, or other fitness institutions. You can find classes of all types in a group setting. Perhaps you love dancing to lose weight—Zumba is a great class for that. Or maybe you like a stationary bike—try a spin class. There is something for everyone. Try out several and pick the ones you like the best.

Ignore the negative

If you find yourself in a group or partnership with people who always want to give up, then you are in the wrong group or partnering with the wrong person. People who think negatively and voice their negative thoughts can depress you and cause you to lose your motivation. You don't want or need that.

You need people who are positive and are just as ready to lose the weight as you are. Surround yourself with people who are ready to lose the weight, get healthy, and do it positively. You can always join a new group or find a new partner if your current support is only discouraging you. If you chose the personal trainer route, don't be afraid to switch trainers too if the one you have isn't clicking with your goals. You will not hurt their feelings—they will have someone else to take your place—but you need to do what's best for you.

If you must change classes or find new partners, just explain that things are not working out the way you had hoped, wish them the best of luck with their weight loss program, and move on. Perhaps you can still keep in touch in some capacity to continue to encourage and motivate each other (perhaps not), but for your ultimate goals to be achieved—do what's best for you.

It is important to love yourself as you are during your weight loss process, no matter how undesirable your weight is to you. Always love yourself inside and out. Always believe in yourself and what you can achieve. No one is perfect, but there is no limit to what you can accomplish if you believe in and love yourself.

If you don't believe in yourself, then certainly no one else will. Always stay true to yourself. Do not worry so much about what others think of you (but pay attention to your friends if they feel you may be going to extremes.).

Always stay positive and think positive. If you think positive, your envisioned outcomes and goals will become more attainable. If you think negatively, then you will have a harder time reaching your goals. Life is too short and hard enough as it is to waste on negativity. Find ways to maintain a positive outlook as you go through this journey.

Learn to ignore the negative things that people throw at you, and work through the negative roadblocks that life naturally throws at you. Learn how to handle negative people and events in a positive manner, even though it will be hard at first.

If your goal is to lose weight, surround yourself with positive people who share or support your goal. Support others in their goals too—sometimes it's easier to give positive advice to a friend than to ourselves, but when speaking those positive things to another person, learn to listen to them for yourself too. Stay focused and driven and, you will thank yourself in the long run.

The Goal Is Achievable

Almost every person who is successful has worked very hard for his or her success. Nothing was easy. Even celebrities, people who seem to have it all, have struggled. They might have started out with some kind of advantage (money, famous parents or a natural ability), but they still had to work hard the rest of the way.

Losing weight will not be easy for you either, but that doesn't mean you have to quit when things get tough and you feel like you're running into a dead end. Remember what they say, "what doesn't kill you will only make you stronger." Other people have done it, are currently doing it, or will begin doing it. The goal is achievable. You can do it.

Once you reach your first milestone, others will come along more easily, and you will find yourself accomplishing your weight loss goal before you know it. It will take time, but with each step closer to your desired weight, you will begin to feel the benefits of losing weight. After losing ten pounds, you may find it easier to take those steps. Perhaps you don't pause at all now on the way up. Or maybe you can take longer walks now without becoming tired. The feeling you will get from reaching those stepping stones will be one of elation and pride at your accomplishment. Use this to motivate yourself to take the next level and reach for your ultimate goal.

I'm sure you have heard many success stories of people who were once overweight and have accomplished their goals of losing the excess weight. You have also probably heard about how hard it was, but they didn't give up. Do you think that if these people struggled that you will not? But if others can do it, then you can too. You can be a success story as well if you keep moving.

Even if you give up, who says you have to be one of the negative statistics? Not me, and anyone who says otherwise is someone you shouldn't be listening to. It's okay to give up for a bit, but get back on the horse before too much time has passed. Give yourself leeway—remember we don't want you to torture yourself. Find ways to re-motivate yourself. Join a support group of women who share your goals. If there aren't groups like that in your area, try forming your own. You can have as many women as you wish in your group, and you can take it to another level by making it an official club. Expand to other areas and cities, wherever you want to go with it. You can help other women lose the weight, get healthy, have fun doing it and keep yourself motivated at the same time! The point is that you want to provide a supportive, caring network for yourself and others.

If forming a group on a large scale or making it official isn't really your thing, you could do a home version and offer your house as a home base, or rotate homes with fellow members. You don't have to register as an official club or group to be one. But find a way to connect with others and get that motivation you all need to keep living the healthy lifestyle. No matter what you do, your focus should ultimately be on losing weight and to reach what is healthy for you. If you can make good friends and connections along the way, then that's even better. One rule to establish: make sure everyone is positive and encouraging to each other. Throughout your weight loss program, take pictures of yourself at various intervals to monitor your progress and encourage yourself to keep on with the diet. You may even find taking your measurements is a good motivational tool as sometimes the inches can come off without it visibly showing.

As you progress and lose weight, share your success with others and assist them with their own weight loss goals. Share tips, recipes, advice and encouragement. You can take your accomplishments as far as you want, and share it with the world if you want to inspire others.

If you think you need to lose weight, or if you want to for health and self-image reasons, get started today. Don't let anything get in your way.

CHAPTER THIRTEEN: NEGATIVE CALORIES AND CARBS = POSITIVE RESULTS?

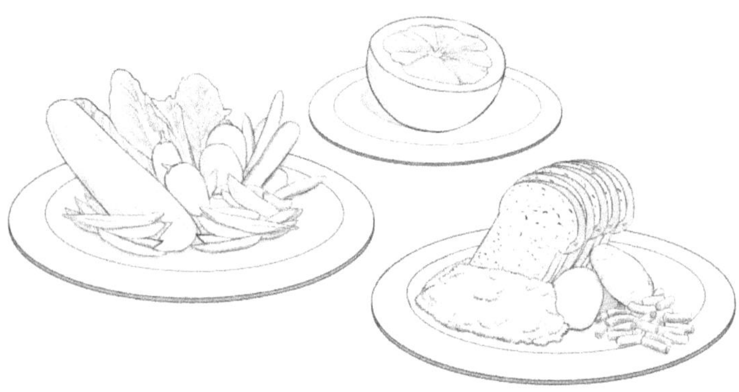

Most people know about the different diets that are out there; but many people don't realize the potential risks of some of these diets. This chapter discusses fad and crash diets. It also exposes the risks and dangers of some diets.

Dieting: Is It Good For You?

Many people believe that they will be happier if they lose a few pounds, drop a couple of dress sizes or tone up. After all, you wouldn't be reading this book if that wasn't true! One of the first things we turn to in our efforts to lose weight is dieting. According to Deanne Jade, Principal of the National Centre for Eating Disorders, in the last ten years 30 % of all adult males and 70% of all adult females have been on a diet at one point or another.

Diets are not a new thing. People have been looking for ways to cut calories and their waistline for centuries. The corset, dating back to the early 1800's was one of the first inventions, still used today, invented to shape our bodies. At the end of the 1800's a man name Horace Fletcher argued that food should be chewed more in order to help aid in weight loss. His diet was termed, "Fletcherizing." But by the early 1900's another diet craze—counting calories—came into focus, leaving Mr. Fletcher's views in the dust. New diets come and go frequently—some good and some not—and each of us need to determine what is best for ourselves and utilize healthy techniques.

Of course, cutting out excess sugar and fat is always a good thing because it leads to a healthier body but some diets take weight loss to extremes and cross a line to where dieting becomes dangerous. Some people believe diets do not work. Their reasoning? If diets worked there wouldn't be so many new one's cropping up every few months and people would not be rushing to try all the new diet products and plans. They believe that strict diets are hard to follow and dieters find it harder to maintain any weight loss.

The truth is diets do work but the results of crash diets and fad diets do not. The key to a successful diet is making it a lifestyle choice—not something that only lasts for a few weeks before moving on to the next diet. When choosing a diet, ensure that you are getting a balanced amount of everything your body craves and needs so that you don't end up binge eating when it becomes too difficult to control your cravings.

New and innovative diets are being designed by people all the time in order to keep up with the demands of people who want to lose weight. It has become a part of the capitalism in America. Many diets are formed for the sole purpose of making money—not to help you lose weight. Therefore, we have a number of different diets at our disposal. Depending upon your body type, lifestyle and nutritional needs you can make the choice about what diet best suits you. But sometimes it's hard to determine which one of the numerous options will suit you best.

Dangers Associated with Crash Dieting

It is important to note that when you choose a diet, do not choose a diet that eliminates most of your food. This is called a "crash diet." Once you start the diet, you will lose weight initially but as soon as you start eating any food again you will put on weight with a vengeance. It is said that the weight you gain post-crash dieting is difficult to shed. Do you really want to take that risk? But weight gain is not the only side effect associated with these dangerous diets.

First, they make you susceptible to psychological and physical illnesses such as Anorexia Nervosa. As we discussed in an earlier chapter, this is where an unhealthy view of one's body begins and people starve themselves in order to stay fit.

Secondly, crash diets do help you lose weight quickly, but they also ensure that you lose lean muscle mass and tissue. Once you lose this lean muscle mass and tissue it results in a decline in your basal metabolic rate, which is the amount of calories your body needs on a daily basis. When your metabolism slows, you'll be more likely to put on weight faster than you did before because your muscle mass is gone.

Lastly, you become weak and prone to several health issues. Crash diets lead to a loss of nutrients in the body causing malnutrition and making the immune system weak. You can also increase your risks for dehydration, heart palpitations and cardiac stress, all unnecessary risks to take just to lose weight quickly.

Low- Carbohydrate diets

These diets restrict or strictly control the intake of carbohydrates in the pursuit of losing weight or for helping treating people with obesity problems. They focus on the consumption of food that contains a higher level of protein and fat as well as allowing food that is low in carbohydrates. They allow consumption of greater portions of nuts and seeds of different kinds, different types of meat and poultry as well as certain vegetables and fruits.

Low-carbohydrate diets will succeed in making or keeping you skinny, and some balanced versions are so beneficial that they are used to treat illnesses such as diabetes, Polycystic Ovarian Syndrome and Chronic Fatigue Syndrome, among others.

If you have ever looked at a glamorous Hollywood celebrity on screen and wished you had a figure like hers, you will be happy to know that one of Hollywood's "worst kept secrets" is that many of the famously skinny actresses are on low-carbohydrate diets. While low-carbohydrate diets have existed for a long time, they burst into popular culture in the 1990's.

If you choose to start a low carb diet, be sure to consult with a doctor on one that is balanced enough to maintain your health. There are many that extremely restrict food intake, causing more health issues.

Fad diets

Fad diets are those that are currently in vogue. They are based usually around one particular food or a combination of certain foods and are easy to follow and very catchy. Very often celebrities go on these diets to lose weight quickly in preparation for movie roles. You may have heard of the Cabbage Soup Diet, the Lemonade Diet or even the South Beach Diet. These are all passing fads that come and go in the diet industry.

Master Cleanse diet

The Master Cleanse Diet is essentially an updated version of a juice fast. This diet does not allow the dieter to consume solid foods at all. It is divided into three parts: drink a cup of herbal tea or a quart of water filled with teaspoons of lemon juice, pepper and honey first thing in the morning. Throughout the day, you can drink up to twelve glasses of lemon drinks and the same herbal tea in the evening. Lemonade is said to help remove excess fat and cleanse the body. This 14-day juice fast has attracted its fair share of followers but has also garnered criticism for being too strict and leading to side effects that show up in the long term. Although it promises to help you lose 20 pounds in just 10 days (how could you not by just drinking liquids?) it can lead to dehydration (because you are basically taking laxatives daily), kidney and other organ issues if used frequently.

The Grapefruit diet

This diet goes as far back as the 1930's America. It focuses on eating grapefruit in large amounts because of the belief that this contains a fat burning enzyme. It is basically a low-carbohydrate diet that says grapefruit must be eaten at every meal along with fat and protein-rich foods because the grapefruit aids in burning the body fat when eaten in combination with these foods. In short, the diet focuses on low-carbohydrate, low-calorie, high-protein food and consumption of grapefruit to aid weight loss. It is mainly a twelve-day plan and can be done repeatedly but 2-day breaks must be given between each cycle.

Although eating grapefruit with other healthy foods is a decent diet choice, the dangers of this diet should be noted. Grapefruit is known to interact with certain medications like statin drugs (like Lipitor), blood pressure medication and allergy drugs so be sure to consult your physician if you are taking any of these medications prior to starting this diet.

The Baby Food diet

This diet had taken Hollywood by storm when it made its debut, but is actually more of a gimmick than a diet. It focuses on adding small containers of baby food into an everyday meal plan in a bid to keep calorie intake in check. Although the "rules" of this fad seem to vary, essentially lower calorie baby food is recommended for one or more meals in a day replacing high calorie meals. Obviously, this would result in weight loss, but baby food can be mushy and unappetizing for many. In addition, you may find yourself utilizing the bathroom a bit more frequently.

Throughout the centuries we have been inundated with the "latest and greatest" fad diets, but in the end, healthy, balanced eating and daily exercise is your best bet. Although utilizing one or more of these fad diets may be okay to help jumpstart your journey, don't rely on them throughout your weight loss routine. Making healthy, daily, choices for the rest of your life will lead to a more satisfied and less tortured way of eating and living. The one thing to remember is that to be thin for your entire life you need to pledge to follow a reasonably balanced diet *forever*, giving your body good quantities without deprivation and allowing for the occasional treat. Stay away from fad and crash diets and then you'll see how a balanced diet can help you facilitate and maintain weight loss.

CHAPTER FOURTEEN: THE SKINNY GIRL DIET

We've come this far, but how can you truly be a Skinny Girl? What does it truly take to achieve this goal?

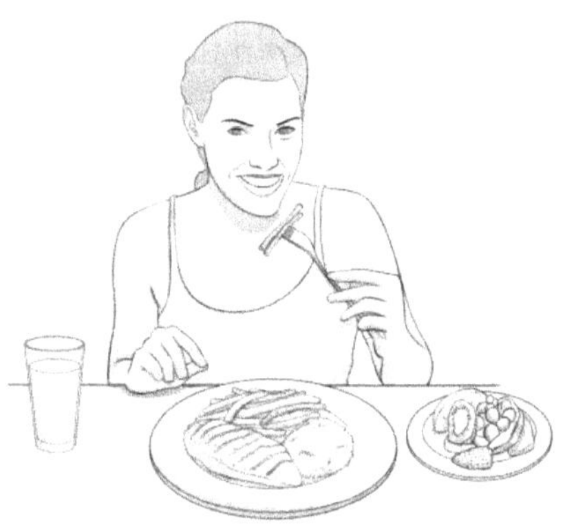

Up until now, we've discussed what we're doing wrong with our diet. We discussed a little about what changes to make and even some recipes to help along the way. But in this final chapter, we'll explore what *right* things to do. To be a skinny girl, you simply have to think like one and eat like one. One of the ways you can do that is by adopting the Skinny Girl Diet.

What is the Skinny Girl Diet?

You might be asking, "What is the Skinny Girl Diet? Is it eating only certain kinds of foods, like a bowl of plain cereal for breakfast, a sandwich for lunch and maybe baked chicken and macaroni and cheese for dinner?" "Is it one of those 'fad' diets that were discussed earlier in this book?" "Is it going to be torturous?"

The answer is, no. It's not those things in any way, shape, form or fashion. Go ahead and toss those thoughts out right now.

The Skinny Girl Diet is thinking, eating and exercising like a skinny girl. It is more than an eating plan, it is a mindset plan as well. It is knowing your ideal, healthy size and working on that goal. You must stick to this diet in a manner that is healthy and satisfying. The Skinny Girl Diet is about focusing on the positive, knowing what you're up against in your quest to get healthier and thinner, and conquering that goal with confidence.

The Skinny Girl Diet consists of any food you can name or think of in the world, even chocolate! It is not limited to certain kinds of foods, but consists of eating foods in a healthy way. It isn't just a dieting plan, but an attitude and philosophy too. Just like thinking positive gets you positive results, thinking skinny will help you become skinny. When your mind is set on achieving that skinny look, you will mentally make choices to obtain that result. That sounds too simple doesn't it?

However, while this plan allows you to eat whatever you want, it is limited in how much food you eat in a single sitting and in one day, depending on how much weight you want to lose (or gain). You should also take into account your recommended caloric intake and your current size. Remember, just because you are skinny doesn't mean you're unhealthy. You can be skinny and unhealthy just like you can be overweight and unhealthy. The purpose of this book and this plan is to help you find that perfect combination of skinny and healthy.

Do you remember what I said at the beginning of this book: "*It's not about what you eat but how much of it you eat.*" That holds true for the Skinny Girl Diet. Eat whatever you want, just eat it in moderation. Incorporate a lot of healthy foods along with exercise. Have that chocolate milkshake you were craving, but have a small one (maybe even just a few sips) for dessert, after a meal of healthy foods. Keep in mind that any extraneous calories you consume that are beyond your recommended amount will come back to haunt you. How much exercise does it take to burn off a small chocolate shake? You might be surprised to know that an 18 ounce chocolate shake would take over an hour on the treadmill—at 6 mph—to burn off. Are you willing to do that just to burn off the shake? (No weight loss here—just to even out the shake's calories.) You have to be able to burn off more calories than you consume each day to lose weight and keep it off. It's really a simple concept after all.

Finding the right diet

I hope everyone who reads this book really think about the message I am trying to send and uses it to assist them with their weight problems. You may find out that you are doing small things that are impeding your weight loss progress. Even if it doesn't apply to you at all, share your new-found knowledge with someone else. We all know someone who is also trying to become a healthier, skinnier person and they may be grateful for the wisdom.

If you are one of the millions of women trying to lose weight, know that it is always best to find and stick with a diet lifestyle that works for you. Find something you are comfortable doing and achieving.

Remember that every diet should involve the following:

1) Eat healthy nutritious foods, as many as you can incorporate daily. Think fruits and vegetables, fish and chicken. Then enjoy your sweets or salty snacks in moderation. Whatever your vice is when it comes to food, don't make that the main focus of your diet. Try to make it a special reward or dessert. It's unhealthy to have that chocolate shake every day, even in small portions. Every once in a while is okay. You must make the effort to include healthy foods in your diet.

2) Moderate your intake, even the healthy stuff. Whether you eat healthy or not, try to eat no more calories than recommended for your size and age, and try to keep the majority of those calories from being "empty." Don't forget that empty calories hold no nutritional value whatsoever (ice cream, candy, and most snack foods like potato chips). This usually makes them the best tasting and the hardest to give up. You don't have to give them up, just eat them in moderation (one or two times a week).

3) Exercise, exercise, exercise. Eating healthier and within the recommended calorie amount is a great start to your diet, but you have to supplement with exercise. Otherwise, it will be harder to lose the weight. If the idea of exercising doesn't appeal to you, try to make the exercise something fun and something you'll enjoy doing. (Refer back to chapter two for some great exercise ideas!) In other words, just get moving. Better yet, get a friend to do it with you. Exercise always seems like less work and more play when you have someone sharing in the activity.

Any diet that does not encourage these key things is not that good of a diet. You will eventually thank yourself when you have reached your goal, when you have finally reached your ideal body weight and done it the natural, healthy way. You will feel a sense of pride for doing it, and this feeling will carry over into other endeavors, as well as be a great starting base to keep the weight off.

Being skinny all my life, I thought the way to being skinny was simple. But when so many people asked me how I achieved it, I knew I had to write this book and share my knowledge with others. Everything I've shared with you is based on my own experiences, theories, opinions and advice on how to lose weight and eat healthier. Just being skinny all my life makes this information real and valuable, but I've also added in important research as well as tools to help you on your journey. If you want to become a skinny girl, you have to eat, and think, like one.

I hope you have learned a lot from this book and I encourage you to share it with others. We can change what is becoming the "obesity norm" in America to one of a healthy girl mindset—one person at a time!

Index

A

B

C

D

E

J

L

M

N

O

P

R

S

T

V

W

Z

www.ingramcontent.com/pod-product-compliance
Lightning Source LLC
Chambersburg PA
CBHW060448280326
41933CB00014B/2703

* 9 7 8 0 6 9 2 5 0 3 0 4 1 *